I0787645

Queen's Divine Balance

The Galveston Diet for Black Women in Menopause

Imani Brooks

Table of Contents

Disclaimer

The information provided in this book, including but not limited to text, graphics, images, and other material, is for informational purposes only. It is not intended as a substitute for professional medical advice, diagnosis, or treatment. Always seek the advice of your physician or other qualified healthcare providers with any questions you may have regarding a medical condition, menopause, or diet, and never disregard professional medical advice or delay seeking it because of something you have read in this book.

The author and publisher of this book are not responsible for any health issues or injuries that may arise from the use or misuse of the information contained in this book. The dietary suggestions and recommendations provided here are based on research and personal experience, but individual results may vary. Every individual's health situation is unique, and it is the responsibility of the reader to consult with their healthcare provider before making any changes to their diet or lifestyle, especially if they have any pre-existing medical conditions.

Neither the author nor the publisher assumes any responsibility or liability for any errors or omissions in the content of this book, nor for any loss, injury, or damage allegedly arising from any information or suggestions in this book.

By reading this book, you acknowledge that you are solely responsible for your own health and well-being, and that the author and publisher are not liable for any direct, indirect, incidental, consequential, or punitive damages resulting from the use of the information in this book.

Introduction

As Black women, we are queens—nurturers, leaders, and warriors in our own right. It's time we reclaim our throne and take the reins on our health, especially during this transformative journey of menopause. Menopause can feel like an uncharted territory where the familiar shifts into new, sometimes challenging experiences. Yet, it also offers a powerful opportunity for growth and self-discovery. This is a call to all Black women to embrace this chapter with grace and power, transforming it into a period of renewal and empowerment.

Menopause marks a significant phase in a woman's life, a transition that is both universal and deeply personal. However, navigating this journey as a Black woman carries unique challenges. Did you know that Black women experience menopause symptoms up to twice as intensely as other demographics? This disparity highlights a critical need for focused dialogue around our experiences and care. Often overlooked in mainstream discussions, our voices and stories must be amplified to ensure that our specific needs are met with understanding and action.

It is essential to recognize that this isn't just about physical changes but also about how we are perceived and treated within healthcare systems. Biases and stereotyping can lead to underdiagnosis and inadequate support, leaving many women feeling isolated during one of the most vulnerable times in their lives. Our collective voices can break through these barriers, demanding better understanding and culturally sensitive care tailored to us. We deserve this attention and respect, and it begins with informing ourselves and each other.

I remember calling my mother one evening, overwhelmed by sudden hot flashes and mood swings. "Welcome to menopause," she laughed, but the tension in her voice revealed the truth: navigating this journey had never come easy for us. My mother's words serve as a reminder that despite generational shifts, the essence of our experiences remains unchanged. Therein lies the beauty and strength; we are connected through shared stories and histories.

This book is not just a guide but a celebration of our resilience. Here, you will find practical strategies, culturally relevant diets, and a roadmap to not just survive menopause, but to thrive during this time. Our approach to food, wellness, and community plays a pivotal role in how we can manage and appreciate the changes unfolding within us. By understanding what fuels our bodies best, we can make informed choices that enhance our well-being, using our rich traditions as a foundation for modern practices.

Throughout history, Black women have borne immense burdens, yet emerged resilient, creating paths where none existed before. For generations, our bodies have carried the weight of historical trauma. Understanding these deeper connections is essential for us to navigate menopause with clarity and strength. The legacy of resilience has been passed down through lines of strong women who have weathered storms both quietly and loudly. This inheritance is part of our identity, fueling our journey through menopause with courage.

As we confront present-day challenges, it's important to see menopause as more than a physical condition—it is a statement of survival, adaptability, and triumph over adversity. The past influences our current experiences, but we have the power to shape our future. We stand on the shoulders of giants, equipped with their wisdom and tenacity, and it's time we leverage this heritage towards crafting vibrant futures for ourselves.

You are not alone on this journey. As we explore this sacred chapter of life together, know that we share the burden, support, and wisdom of one another—just as our foremothers did before us. In these pages, you will discover not only guidance but community. Let us forge a sisterhood of solidarity, where knowledge and empathy unite us, strengthening our resolve to live fully and fearlessly.

To the health professionals and caregivers reading, your role in this journey is invaluable. To truly support the Black women in your care, understanding their specific needs and experiences is crucial. This book offers insights and tools to help bridge gaps and foster environments where informed and empathetic treatment flourishes. Your awareness and advocacy can transform lives, creating lasting impacts that extend beyond individual care.

For wellness coaches and nutritionists, here lies an opportunity to expand your expertise in culturally appropriate dietary strategies. Menopause is a multifaceted experience that benefits from holistic approaches. By incorporating cultural relevance into wellness practices, you are empowering and equipping women with knowledge that resonates with their lived realities. Together, we can redefine wellness standards, ensuring they reflect and respect diversity.

In conclusion, this book invites every reader to embark on a journey of empowerment, enlightenment, and transformation. Menopausing as a Black woman can indeed be an enriching experience when approached with confidence and community. With awareness and supportive resources, this transitional phase becomes not just manageable, but a testament to enduring strength and beauty.

Our shared stories weave together the fabric of resilience, forming a tapestry of hope and understanding. Let us move forward with united hearts and minds, embracing this chapter with open arms and fierce determination. Together, we can turn the tide, creating a menopause narrative that honors and uplifts every Black woman on her path to greatness.

Chapter 1: Reclaiming Your Royal Power

Reclaiming your royal power during menopause is about embracing a transformative phase where you can reign over your own well-being. Menopause, while universal, often presents unique challenges for Black women, influenced by cultural, social, and economic factors. These nuances can make the journey through menopause feel isolating and complex. Yet, it is precisely within these challenges that there lies an opportunity for empowerment and self-discovery. By understanding and valuing these distinct experiences, Black women are positioned not as silent sufferers but as queens, commanding control over their health and embracing the natural transitions their bodies undergo.

In this chapter, we delve deeply into the specifics of how menopause uniquely impacts Black women. You will explore the varied symptoms that may manifest differently in Black women, along with the cultural influences that shape these experiences. The chapter highlights the importance of recognizing these differences and adapting healthcare strategies accordingly. Additionally, the narrative will guide readers through the relevance of culturally tailored wellness practices, emphasizing the role of community support and shared knowledge. This approach not only aims to provide relief from menopausal symptoms but also to empower Black women to assert their agency, reclaim their narratives, and celebrate their strength during this pivotal life stage.

Overview of Menopause and Its Impact on Black Women

Menopause is a natural and inevitable phase of life, marking the end of menstrual cycles. It's often characterized by symptoms such as hot flashes, mood swings, night sweats, and sleep disturbances. For many women, these experiences can be disruptive and challenging as they navigate this significant transition. While menopause is a shared biological process among all women, there are nuances and distinctive challenges that Black women encounter during this period.

The mainstream discussions about menopause generally aim to address universal symptoms and remedies, yet often fail to incorporate the unique perspectives and needs of Black women. This oversight can lead to feelings of alienation and neglect, as if their experiences are invisible or deemed insignificant compared to the broader population. In truth, Black women's menopausal journeys are colored by not just the general symptoms but also cultural, social, and economic factors that influence their health outcomes.

It is crucial to highlight how certain symptoms might manifest differently in Black women compared to what is typically described in generalized health literature. For example, research suggests that Black women may experience more intense vasomotor symptoms, such as more frequent and severe hot flashes, than other racial groups. Additionally, Black women may encounter menopause-related changes earlier and possibly for a longer duration.

Recognizing these deviations is necessary because it underscores the fact that one-size-fits-all descriptions do not suffice. Menopause is deeply personal, and culture and ethnicity play a significant role in shaping the experience. By acknowledging these differences, we can better address the specific needs and challenges faced by

Black women, thereby empowering them to claim agency over their health.

This recognition leads to the next pivotal point: the need for tailored health strategies that cater specifically to Black women. Health professionals, caregivers, and wellness practitioners must consider the particularities of Black women's experiences when devising support plans. This involves more than just adapting known solutions; it requires an understanding of cultural influences, accessibility issues, and trust dynamics between Black women and medical institutions.

For healthcare providers, this means engaging with Black communities to gain insight into lived experiences and building trust through culturally sensitive care. It involves creating spaces where Black women feel safe and heard, reinforcing that their unique menopausal experiences matter. Culturally relevant education about menopause should be offered, integrating traditional knowledge and modern insights to bridge any gaps.

At the same time, wellness coaches and nutritionists can play a crucial role by developing dietary practices that acknowledge cultural preferences while promoting health and well-being. Emphasizing traditional foods within Black culture while incorporating beneficial nutritional advice can make a positive difference. This approach values the deep-rooted connections between food, identity, and health, providing guidance that resonates personally with individuals seeking to manage their menopausal symptoms in a holistic manner.

Furthermore, deploying supportive community networks can bolster these individualized strategies. Community centers, online forums, and local events create supportive environments where Black women can share their experiences, obtain valuable advice, and foster empowerment. Encouraging communal engagement not only offers practical support but also reinforces a collective strength that can be particularly beneficial in navigating the physical and emotional layers of menopause.

Importantly, addressing these needs goes beyond providing immediate relief from symptoms. It's about empowering Black women to reclaim their royal power during menopause, elevating them as queens who are informed and confident in managing their health. When health narratives include and embrace the diversity of Black women's experiences, it opens the door to more equitable and effective care.

By championing tailored approaches, we shift the narrative from a prescriptive model to one that celebrates individuality and acknowledges the distinct journeys of Black women. Ultimately, recognizing the multi-dimensionality of menopause and its impact enables us to offer more comprehensive, nuanced support—where each woman's experience is validated and addressed with compassion and precision.

Historical Narratives Affecting Black Women's Health

The history of health narratives for Black women has been shaped by a myriad of cultural, social, and political influences. To reclaim their agency and control over health, particularly during menopause, an understanding of this past is crucial. Traditionally, within the Black community, beliefs about female health have often intertwined with broader social roles. For instance, the archetype of the "strong Black woman" has historically dictated that Black women must be resilient and self-reliant, often at the expense of their well-being. This perception can lead to underreporting of health issues or reluctance to seek medical help, reinforcing a cycle where needs are overshadowed by expectations.

Historically, Black women's activism has made significant strides in challenging these narrations. Some key figures, like Fannie Lou Hamer and Mary Eliza Mahoney, paved the way for better health outcomes through advocacy and professional success. Fannie Lou Hamer, known for her civil rights activism, also spotlighted health injustices faced by Black women, such as non-consensual sterilizations under government programs. Her efforts have laid a foundation for demanding health rights and systemic change. Similarly, Mary Eliza Mahoney, the first African American professionally trained nurse, broke racial barriers and inspired generations of Black women to enter the medical field, thus increasing representation and influence on health care services. Their stories highlight how activism can serve as a powerful tool in reframing health narratives.

Despite these advances, the rhetoric surrounding strength continues to suppress health needs in contemporary times. The expectation to embody resilience may cause hesitation in expressing vulnerability or seeking assistance when dealing with menopausal symptoms. Strength has become a double-edged sword, providing empowerment while also imposing silence. Women might feel compelled to endure discomfort without complaint, perpetuating a narrative that neglects the importance of addressing personal health concerns.

Encouraging self-reflection can be an effective way to redefine these personal health narratives using historical knowledge. By analyzing past hardships and victories, Black women can identify patterns of suppression in their health management and choose pathways that prioritize well-being. For example, reflecting on the legacies of activists reminds us that advocating for personal rights is not only permissible but essential. Recognizing that vulnerability does not equate to weakness allows for more open conversations about health needs.

Moreover, embracing one's history enables a reclamation of agency. Understanding how past movements fought for rights empowers modern women to demand appropriate healthcare tailored to their unique experiences during menopause. Engaging with supportive communities or networks provides shared histories and collective encouragement. These groups can facilitate exchanges of culturally relevant health strategies, ensuring decisions are informed and holistic.

Additionally, it's paramount to address the lack of inclusive research in medicine. Despite increasing awareness, gaps remain in understanding how menopause uniquely affects Black women due to generalized studies predominantly focusing on white populations. Advocacy for more inclusive research can ensure that future medical literature accurately reflects diverse menopausal experiences. Such efforts would likely lead to more personalized healthcare options, ultimately allowing Black women greater control over their health journeys.

The need for advocacy cannot be overstated, and it extends beyond individual actions. Health professionals, caregivers, wellness coaches, and nutritionists all have roles to play in dismantling outdated perceptions and contributing towards more equitable health frameworks. They can educate themselves on the specific needs of Black women during menopause, offering support that acknowledges both challenges and strengths born from cultural heritage.

Understanding these dynamics equips readers to challenge historical narratives and reclaim agency. This approach doesn't merely aim to inform; it seeks to empower. In a world where marginalized voices have too often been overlooked, seizing control over one's health narrative becomes a radical act of self-empowerment and societal transformation.

Setting the Empowering Tone of the Book

In the grand tapestry of history, Black women have repeatedly demonstrated a remarkable resilience. From overcoming societal challenges to thriving amidst adversity, their strength is woven through narratives that span generations. This subpoint aims to celebrate this incredible fortitude and affirm it during the transformative phase of menopause. Often, these stories are not given the spotlight they deserve, yet they hold an immense power to inspire. Consider the stories of women like Harriet Tubman and Rosa Parks who defied odds and overcame monumental hurdles. Their legacies remind us that Black women have always harnessed a deep-seated strength to lead and empower themselves and others.

Menopause, a natural phase in a woman's life, can sometimes feel daunting. It brings with it changes and challenges that might seem overwhelming. Yet, it's also an opportunity to reclaim control over one's health and well-being. This book serves as a resource, offering valuable insights and fostering a supportive environment where understanding thrives. By nurturing this understanding, we encourage Black women to view menopause not as a loss but as a new chapter ripe with potential for growth and empowerment. It's about creating a community where shared experiences lay the foundation for support, reminding every Black woman that she is not alone on this journey.

Fostering a positive outlook is essential. It's easy to become ensnared in focusing solely on the obstacles presented by menopause. Still, it's crucial to remember what can be achieved despite them. Recognizing small triumphs—whether it's mastering a new wellness routine or simply embracing a day with energy and vigor—can serve as powerful motivators. Celebrating these victories reinforces positivity and builds momentum, encouraging a mindset shift from merely enduring menopause to thriving through it.

Furthermore, inspiring action and change involves recognizing the importance of proactive management. Taking charge of one's health through informed lifestyle choices and clear communication with healthcare providers is vital. This proactive stance doesn't just stop at personal benefit; it amplifies collective empowerment. When Black women take ownership of their menopausal journey, they set an example for peers, subsequently igniting a chain reaction of empowerment throughout the community. Sharing insights and resources spreads knowledge, underscoring the collective ability to support one another.

Understanding menopause better facilitates improved quality of life, so it's important to bridge awareness and practical strategies. Guidelines suggest exploring dietary choices, physical activity, and mindfulness practices tailored to meet individual needs. Education about menopause is a powerful tool; it can demystify common misconceptions and highlight effective coping mechanisms. By framing menopause within the context of empowerment, women are encouraged to embrace this phase as part of their identity—not a deviation from it.

Community perspectives add depth to this narrative. The collective voice of Black women experiencing menopause echoes louder when amplified together. Encouraging conversations in safe spaces—be it community groups, online forums, or casual gatherings—fosters solidarity and mutual support. Beyond sharing challenges, these interactions reveal solutions rooted in cultural understanding and lived experience. They act as reminders that while each journey is unique, the bonds formed around shared experiences offer immeasurable strength.

Introduction to Cultural Dietary Practices

Within the intricate tapestry of Black culture, food serves not only as sustenance but also as a powerful expression of identity and heritage. Understanding the roots of dietary choices is essential for Black women navigating menopause, a time when health and well-being are paramount. Throughout history, traditional foods have been deeply embedded in cultural practices, offering both nutritional value and comfort. Collard greens, yams, black-eyed peas, and millet are more than just ingredients; they symbolize endurance, community, and connection to ancestry. These foods carry stories of resilience from generations past, forming an integral part of a health journey that embraces the essence of who we are.

Merging these traditional foods with modern nutritional insights can unlock new pathways to wellness during menopause. For instance, black-eyed peas are rich in fiber and protein, supporting digestive health and providing sustained energy levels. Yams contain diosgenin, a natural compound that may help regulate hormonal balance. When combined with modern understanding, such as incorporating omega-3 rich fish or seeds like flaxseed, the benefits are amplified. This fusion not only enriches the diet but also grounds it in tradition while adapting to contemporary needs. Embracing this approach empowers Black women to navigate menopause with confidence, balancing the wisdom of ancestors with current scientific knowledge.

Integrating cultural practices into modern wellness approaches goes beyond honoring traditions; it revitalizes them. Consider incorporating rituals around meal preparation and consumption, which can foster mindfulness and community. Practices like communal cooking and shared family meals provide social support, crucial for emotional well-being during menopause. Incorporating spice-rich sauces not only enhances flavor but can also provide anti-inflammatory benefits, aiding in managing menopausal symptoms like joint pain. By reshaping how these practices fit within busy lives, we make space for cultural richness in everyday routines. This holistic integration emphasizes that wellness doesn't have to be an isolated pursuit but is entwined with shared experiences and collective healing.

Practical applications of these principles can be effortless yet transformative. Start by including more plant-based ingredients that are staples in Black cuisine. A weekly menu might feature dishes like okra stew or coconut rice, celebrating both taste and nutrition. Reducing processed elements and focusing on whole foods paves the way for improved health outcomes. For those new to certain traditional foods, simple methods like roasting or steaming can reveal their flavors without overwhelming the palate. Encouraging experimentation with herbs and spices commonly used in African and Caribbean dishes—such as turmeric, thyme, and ginger—can offer additional health benefits, including anti-aging properties.

Beyond individual meal planning, there's strength in community initiatives that prioritize cultural food education. Cooking workshops and classes tailored toward Black women can rejuvenate interest in traditional recipes while highlighting their nutritional advantages. These gatherings become spaces for shared learning and mutual support, allowing participants to swap advice and inspire one another. Moreover, advocating for access to culturally relevant foods in local markets ensures that healthy choices are practical and accessible. Community gardens offer another avenue, providing fresh produce while fostering a deeper connection to food sources and environmental stewardship.

Another dimension of incorporating cultural foods into daily life involves creating a supportive environment at home. Encourage family members to engage with traditions, whether through celebrating specific culinary customs or exploring the history behind favorite dishes. This involvement not only enriches the family's collective experience but nurtures a sense of pride in cultural heritage. Within this setting, children learn the importance of these foods early on, laying the groundwork for lifelong healthy eating habits. Additionally, sharing personal stories about how certain meals evoke memories or emotions can strengthen familial bonds and cultivate a positive atmosphere around dining.

Health professionals and caregivers play a pivotal role in this cultural reclamation during menopause. By recognizing the importance of culturally relevant dietary practices, they can offer advice that resonates on a personal level. Tailoring dietary recommendations to include familiar foods encourages adherence and success in managing menopausal symptoms. Nutritionists and wellness coaches should seek to understand traditional diets, emphasizing their benefits alongside modern nutrition science. This culturally sensitive approach not only validates emotional connections to food but positions these practices as valuable allies in achieving optimal health.

The Promise of Self-Empowerment and Wellness

Menopause is a significant life phase that requires careful navigation and informed decisions, especially for

Black women stepping into this period. Embracing the idea of being a queen in control of your health during menopause involves actively taking part in your healthcare journey. This begins with informed decision-making. Arming yourself with knowledge about menopause will empower you to make choices that align with your personal needs and preferences. Instead of being a passive participant, engage proactively by asking questions and seeking out information from trusted health professionals. Ensure that your healthcare provider understands your specific concerns and cultural context, which can significantly impact the care you receive.

To truly reclaim power during menopause, it is essential to understand resilience not just as enduring hardships but as a dynamic process of growth. Resilience stems from effective coping strategies. Adopting healthy habits such as regular exercise, balanced nutrition, and adequate sleep can be instrumental in building resilience. These practices not only help manage physical symptoms like hot flashes and joint pain, but they also support mental well-being. Mindfulness and stress-reduction techniques, such as yoga and meditation, are powerful tools to foster inner strength. They enable you to approach challenges with a positive mindset, turning potential setbacks into opportunities for growth.

A comprehensive approach to health during menopause integrates mental, emotional, and physical well-being. It is crucial not to consider these aspects in isolation but as interconnected components of overall health. Pay attention to mental health by addressing feelings of anxiety or depression that may arise during this transition. Emotional wellness should not be overlooked; acknowledging and communicating your feelings is vital. Physical health goes beyond managing symptoms—it encompasses maintaining an active lifestyle and a nutritious diet tailored to your unique needs. By considering all these facets together, you create a holistic health strategy that empowers you in every aspect of life.

Connecting with your community can greatly enhance this journey. Building and relying on communal ties provides shared support and understanding. Engage in conversations with other Black women who are experiencing similar transitions. Their insights and experiences can offer comfort and practical tips. Community gatherings or support groups can serve as safe spaces for sharing stories and solutions, reducing feelings of isolation. Strengthening these connections fortifies a network that contributes to enhanced well-being, reminding you that you are not alone in this journey.

Guidelines for creating a safe space within your community can aid in fostering genuine connection and support. Begin by establishing an open dialogue where everyone feels heard and valued. Encourage members to share their experiences without judgment. Promote inclusivity by welcoming diverse perspectives and backgrounds. Facilitate activities focused on stress relief and encouragement, such as group yoga sessions or cooking classes centered around nutritious meals for menopause. When community members feel safe and supported, they empower each other through shared knowledge and camaraderie.

Another key aspect is embracing positivity throughout this journey. Focus on the potential for personal transformation that menopause brings. Incorporating daily affirmations can reinforce a positive self-image and instill confidence. Celebrate the small victories along the way—whether it's incorporating a new healthy routine or successfully managing a challenging symptom. Positivity is contagious; by adopting an optimistic outlook, you inspire others to see menopause as a transition filled with possibilities rather than limitations.

Manifesting change involves setting realistic goals for your menopause journey. Start by clearly identifying what you wish to achieve, whether it's improved physical health, better emotional balance, or enriched community ties. Break these objectives into smaller, manageable steps. For example, if you're aiming for better fitness, begin with short, daily walks and gradually increase intensity and duration. Regularly review and adjust your goals as needed, allowing flexibility to accommodate changes in your circumstances or priorities. Tracking progress not only keeps you motivated but also helps recognize the progress you've made—a testament to your resilience and capability.

As you embark on this empowering journey, remember to incorporate feedback from those who support and care for you. Open discussions with caregivers and health professionals can provide valuable insights and alternative viewpoints. Sharing your experiences and aspirations enables them to tailor their support more effectively. This collaboration enriches your path by integrating external perspectives with your personal needs, further solidifying your sense of control and empowerment.

Concluding Thoughts

In this chapter, we've explored the journey of menopause from the perspective of Black women, positioning them as empowered individuals who can navigate health and well-being like royalty. We discussed how the experience of menopause is unique for Black women, shaped by cultural, social, and historical factors. By acknowledging these differences, we stress the importance of tailored health strategies that resonate with their lived experiences. The goal is to shift the narrative from one-size-fits-all solutions to approaches that celebrate individuality and cultural richness, ensuring that each woman feels seen, heard, and supported.

As we conclude, remember that reclaiming agency over one's health during menopause is not just a possibility but a reality within reach. Whether you are seeking guidance as a Black woman experiencing menopause, a health professional aiming to provide more inclusive care, or a wellness coach developing culturally relevant strategies, we encourage you to embrace this journey with confidence and determination. Building supportive networks and fostering positive community engagement can further enhance this empowerment, transforming menopause into an opportunity for growth. By integrating traditional practices with modern insights, we create a comprehensive framework for thriving, celebrating strength, resilience, and the unique heritage of Black women.

Chapter 2: Navigating Unique Menopause Journeys

Cultural and Genetic Influences on Menopause Among Black Women

Menopause among Black women is a complex journey influenced by various intertwining factors. This chapter delves into how history, socio-economic conditions, and cultural narratives uniquely shape the menopausal experience for Black women. The collective weight of historical trauma, enduring through generations, manifests in ways that impact hormonal balance, often making menopause symptoms more challenging to manage. This exploration highlights the resilience and strength embedded within cultural practices, which offer necessary emotional support and a sense of community, counteracting the stressors faced during this transition.

Throughout this chapter, you will gain insight into how historical stressors have persisted and influenced menopause symptoms among Black women, emphasizing the link between chronic stress and hormonal imbalances. Discussions include examining socio-economic barriers like healthcare access, nutrition, and education which further exacerbate health disparities. In addressing these aspects, the chapter also points to the transformative power of community support systems, from local networks to spiritual spaces, providing both psychological relief and practical coping mechanisms. Furthermore, there's a focus on the critical role of mental health care, advocating for holistic approaches that integrate physical, mental, and spiritual well-being. By navigating these layered experiences, the chapter encourages readers—whether experiencing menopause or supporting those who are—to recognize the necessity of culturally sensitive strategies in managing menopause health challenges effectively.

Impact of Historical Stress on Menopause Symptoms

Navigating the journey of menopause can be uniquely challenging for Black women, as it is intricately linked to both cultural and genetic influences. Historical stressors and their lingering effects serve as a lens through which we can better understand these experiences. Chronic stress from historical trauma has often resulted in hormonal imbalances that make menopause symptoms more severe or difficult to manage. The impact of such trauma is deeply rooted in history, with its origins in systemic inequities that have persisted over generations.

Black women have faced numerous challenges due to the enduring legacy of slavery, segregation, and racial discrimination. These historical stressors do not merely reside in the past; they echo into the present, manifesting as chronic stress. Stress activates the body's hormonal response, impairing the balance necessary for smooth menopausal transition. This imbalance can lead to more intense hot flashes, night sweats, mood swings, and other common menopause symptoms. Studies highlight the link between stress and the disruption of hormones like cortisol, estrogen, and progesterone—key players in menopause regulation.

Systemic inequities further exacerbate these health disparities among Black women during menopause. Inequitable access to healthcare, quality nutrition, and education consistently hinders effective management of menopause symptoms. Such disparities are not accidental but are reflective of broader social and economic inequities that disproportionately affect Black communities. Limited resources mean that many Black women have less opportunity to seek specialized care or to access culturally sensitive health guidance, hindering their ability to find appropriate solutions during this life stage.

Despite these hurdles, resilience embedded in cultural practices provides a powerful source of emotional support. Traditions, community networks, and culturally significant rituals contribute positively by offering psychological reprieve and a sense of belonging. For instance, the collective experience shared within African American churches or family gatherings can provide comfort and solidarity. The strength found in these communal spaces helps to counterbalance the stressors and offer emotional sustenance during challenging times.

The importance of mental health in managing menopause symptoms cannot be overstated, and addressing it requires recognizing the need for holistic approaches. Incorporating mental, physical, and spiritual care into one's lifestyle allows for a comprehensive strategy that not only addresses symptoms but also fosters overall well-being. By focusing on self-care techniques such as yoga, meditation, and mindfulness practices, Black women can mitigate the negative impacts of stress on their bodies. Physical activities tailored to individual preferences, like dance or walking, can further enhance physical health while providing joy and relaxation.

Guidelines empowering readers to address their mental health highlight the value of seeking therapy or counseling, particularly when dealing with unresolved trauma or current stressors. Understanding the profound effect that mental wellness has on physical symptoms enables a proactive approach to holistic care. Additionally, utilizing community resources such as support groups or faith-based counseling services can offer personalized support in navigating menopause.

Community resources for mental wellness hold tremendous potential in empowering Black women during menopause. Engaging with peers facing similar challenges offers an opportunity for shared learning, encouragement, and collective healing. Group therapy or talking circles create safe spaces where women can express themselves freely, exchange coping strategies, and draw strength from communal bonds. Accessing culturally competent professionals who appreciate the unique factors influencing their menopause experience further enriches this support system.

Socio-economic Influences on Health Outcomes

Socio-economic status significantly impacts the menopause experience for Black women, influencing factors such as access to healthcare, nutrition, education, and employment stress. Understanding these dynamics can help individuals and professionals provide better support and resources tailored to this group's unique needs.

One primary way socio-economic status affects menopause is through access to healthcare. Limited healthcare resources impact access to necessary treatments, screenings, and advice essential during menopause. Many Black women face obstacles in obtaining affordable healthcare, which can lead to inadequate management of menopause symptoms like hot flashes, mood swings, and sleep disorders. Healthcare facilities in lower-income neighborhoods often lack specialized practitioners or comprehensive services, making it harder for women to receive accurate diagnoses or effective treatment plans. Consequently, a critical understanding of how to navigate healthcare systems becomes invaluable. Encouraging self-reflection on personal and familial experiences can empower women to prioritize their health despite these challenges. One guideline could be cultivating awareness of community health resources and developing relationships with supportive healthcare providers, both of which are vital steps toward improved menopause care.

Financial constraints further complicate the situation by limiting access to nutritious foods crucial for managing menopause symptoms. Proper nutrition plays a key role in alleviating symptoms like weight gain and bone density loss. Yet, healthier food options can often be more expensive or less readily available in predominantly Black neighborhoods. The prevalence of food deserts—areas with limited access to grocery stores or fresh produce—restricts dietary choices, potentially leading to nutrient deficiencies that exacerbate menopause symptoms. A diet lacking in calcium, vitamin D, and other vital nutrients can have lasting impacts on overall health during menopause. Encouraging initiatives like community gardens, local farmers' markets, and nutritional education programs can make a difference. These not only enhance access to healthier foods but also foster community engagement and empowerment.

Education level also plays a significant role in shaping the menopause experience. Health literacy is pivotal when it comes to understanding menopause symptoms and making informed decisions about treatment options. Individuals with higher education levels may be more likely to research symptoms, seek out professional advice, or engage in preventative health measures. Unfortunately, systemic inequities in educational opportunities mean that many women of lower socio-economic status might not possess the same health literacy, potentially delaying diagnosis and treatment for menopause-related issues. Educational workshops and accessible literature specifically addressing menopause in the context of the Black woman's experience could promote better health outcomes. By enhancing health literacy, these resources empower women to take control of their well-being.

Employment stress adds another layer of complexity to the menopause experience among Black women. High-stress work environments, often coupled with discrimination or job insecurity, can amplify menopause symptoms. Stress is known to contribute significantly to hormonal imbalances, intensifying symptoms such as anxiety, irritability, and fatigue. This can become a vicious cycle—menopause symptoms affecting work performance, leading to increased stress, which then worsens the symptoms. Developing workplace policies that acknowledge and accommodate the menopause experience is crucial. Flexible working hours, wellness programs, and supportive supervisors can help mitigate stress and improve quality of life during this transitional phase.

Furthermore, advocating for acknowledging historical impacts in individual health narratives offers an additional perspective. Societal structures and historical contexts have long influenced health inequities experienced by Black women. Recognizing these influences provides deeper insight into how socio-economic factors shape health outcomes. Addressing these broader systemic issues requires collective community efforts and advocacy for policy changes.

Diverse Symptom Presentation Among Black Women

Menopause is an inevitable phase in every woman's life, yet its manifestation can vary widely among individuals. For Black women, these variations are often more pronounced due to a range of cultural, genetic, and socio-economic factors. Menopause symptoms, as traditionally described in medical literature, may not always align with the experiences of Black women. This discrepancy highlights the need for personalized healthcare approaches that take into account the unique attributes and challenges faced by this demographic.

One of the key issues is the broad spectrum of symptoms that go beyond the common complaints of hot flashes and night sweats. Many Black women report experiencing menopause differently, with symptoms that might not be highlighted in mainstream medical discussions. These can include severe joint pain, mood fluctuations, and unusual skin changes. Such differences underscore the importance of recognizing that menopause is not a one-size-fits-all experience, especially when it comes to Black women whose experiences have been underrepresented in research and medical narratives.

Psychological symptoms also play a significant role during menopause, with anxiety being particularly prevalent among Black women. The pressures stemming from both internal physiological changes and external societal expectations can exacerbate anxiety levels. Recognizing these psychological aspects is crucial because they can profoundly affect quality of life and overall well-being. Anxiety during menopause may manifest as increased worry, irritability, or even panic attacks, necessitating tailored therapeutic interventions. Health professionals need to be vigilant in addressing these symptoms, offering supportive counseling and appropriate therapies to help manage psychological challenges effectively.

Cultural perspectives further influence how physical changes during menopause are perceived and managed. Cultural beliefs and values shape how symptoms are interpreted and what responses they elicit. For many

Black women, community support and shared cultural understandings provide a vital framework for navigating menopause. Traditional remedies or holistic practices, often passed down through generations, are frequently employed alongside or instead of conventional medical treatments. Understanding these cultural contexts is essential for healthcare providers who aim to offer respectful and relevant care options.

In particular, reinforcing the significance of cultural connections in healing can aid in symptom management. For instance, storytelling and sharing personal experiences within community settings can serve as powerful tools for empowerment and coping. These activities foster a sense of belonging and mutual understanding while also providing practical advice and emotional support. Encouraging participation in community support groups can therefore be highly beneficial, offering spaces where Black women can voice their concerns and gain strength from collective wisdom.

Improved communication with healthcare providers is another critical factor that enhances symptom management during menopause. Open and honest dialogue builds trust and facilitates the exchange of necessary information. However, achieving this can be challenging due to potential mismatches in cultural understandings and communication styles between patients and providers. Training healthcare professionals in cultural competence can bridge these gaps, ensuring that interactions are respectful and productive. By actively listening and validating their experiences, health practitioners can help Black women feel seen and heard, ultimately leading to more effective symptom management strategies.

Moreover, empowering Black women to advocate for their own needs within the healthcare system can yield better outcomes. Educating women about possible symptoms and treatment options allows them to make informed decisions and ask pertinent questions. They should feel encouraged to express their preferences regarding treatments, whether they lean towards lifestyle adjustments, natural remedies, or medical interventions. Healthcare providers can guide this process by presenting various options and respecting the individual choices of their patients.

Need for Increased Representation in Research

The journey of menopause is a deeply personal experience, differing widely not just in symptoms but also in cultural context. Black women have historically been underrepresented in menopause research, leading to gaps in understanding their unique experiences and needs. This lack of diversity in research is problematic as it deprives both healthcare providers and Black women themselves of comprehensive insights necessary for effective health management. The cultural nuances and genetic factors distinct to Black women are often glossed over, with most studies centered around predominantly white populations. As such, these studies may not accurately reflect or address the specific challenges faced by Black women during menopause.

By prioritizing diverse representation, research can better capture the full spectrum of menopause experiences. Community-based research models offer a significant advantage here. Such approaches involve engaging directly with communities to gather data that reflects real-world settings and lived experiences. By diving into the community, researchers can unravel stories and insights that laboratory settings might miss. When researchers listen to and learn from participants, they gain a richer, more nuanced understanding of how menopause manifests differently across various demographics. For instance, exploring the impact of cultural perceptions on health-related behaviors can shed light on why Black women may respond differently to certain symptoms or treatments.

Cultural competence in research design is crucial to achieving meaningful outcomes. Researchers who understand the cultural contexts of their subjects can tailor their methodologies and questions accordingly. This involves respecting beliefs, traditions, and social dynamics unique to Black women's communities. Culturally competent research not only improves the accuracy of findings but also enhances participant trust and engagement. Trust is a vital component, especially given historical mistrust between Black communities and medical institutions. When participants feel their culture is respected and valued in research, they are more likely to engage openly and share their experiences honestly.

Knowledge sharing stemming from research is another vital aspect. The insights gained through inclusive studies must be disseminated back into the communities from where they emerged. Women armed with accurate information about menopause are empowered to advocate for their health needs effectively. They can make informed decisions about their treatment options and lifestyle changes and feel confident to voice concerns in healthcare settings. Advocacy becomes a natural extension of knowledge, helping women navigate health systems that may not always recognize or prioritize their needs.

Community workshops and support groups can be wonderful platforms for sharing research findings. They provide safe spaces for women to not only receive information but also discuss their experiences and learn from one another. This exchange of knowledge can foster a sense of community and solidarity among Black women, reassuring them that they are not alone in their journey. It also encourages intergenerational dialogue, where older women can pass down wisdom and coping strategies to younger generations facing menopause.

For healthcare professionals and caregivers aiming to support Black women effectively, understanding the nuances uncovered by diverse research is key. It equips them with the perspectives needed to offer culturally sensitive care and create an environment of inclusivity within healthcare settings. Health professionals who are aware of the specific challenges faced by Black women can develop tailored treatment plans that respect cultural practices while addressing medical needs.

Furthermore, wellness coaches and nutritionists can utilize this knowledge to recommend culturally relevant dietary strategies and wellness practices. These personalized approaches not only improve physical well-being but also resonate emotionally with clients, enhancing adherence and satisfaction with the care received. By acknowledging and incorporating cultural strengths and preferences, wellness practices become more holistic and impactful.

Challenges and Opportunities for Advocacy

Advocacy for Black women experiencing menopause presents unique challenges and opportunities, deeply rooted in both cultural stereotypes and the healthcare system's complexities. Cultural stereotypes often pose significant barriers to effective health advocacy, shaping perceptions and interactions with healthcare providers. These stereotypes may lead some professionals to make assumptions about Black women's health needs, potentially resulting in miscommunication or inadequate care. For instance, there's a stereotype that Black women are strong and can tolerate more pain, which might affect how their symptoms are validated and treated. This highlights the necessity of breaking down these stereotypes through education and awareness, ensuring healthcare providers approach each case with fresh eyes and without preconceived notions.

Equipping Black women with skills to navigate healthcare systems is essential for achieving better health outcomes during menopause. Understanding how to effectively communicate with healthcare providers, what questions to ask, and when to seek second opinions can empower women to take control of their health journeys. Many resources, such as workshops and online courses, aim to enhance these skills. Encouraging proactive engagement in one's healthcare not only fosters individual empowerment but can also instigate broader systemic changes as informed patients demand better and more inclusive care.

Leveraging community resources plays a pivotal role in increasing awareness and support for Black women during menopause. Community centers, local health organizations, and support groups provide safe spaces for sharing experiences and receiving guidance. These resources often offer culturally relevant information and strategies that resonate more deeply than generalized advice. For example, local wellness programs might incorporate traditional dietary practices or natural remedies familiar to Black women, making recommendations more accessible and relatable. By tapping into these community assets, women can find both empowerment and practical solutions tailored to their specific needs.

Sharing knowledge within peer groups is another powerful way to strengthen advocacy efforts among Black women. Peer groups provide vital emotional support and an exchange of personal experiences, fostering a collective wisdom that formal healthcare settings sometimes overlook. In these circles, members can learn from others' successes and setbacks, gaining insights into managing symptoms and navigating healthcare systems. Moreover, these groups can serve as catalysts for change, as shared experiences highlight common challenges that can be addressed collectively through advocacy and activism. Building networks of informed individuals amplifies voices that often go unheard in larger healthcare conversations, pushing for necessary reforms and acknowledgment of diverse menopause experiences.

In urging readers to be proactive in seeking out healthcare opportunities, it's crucial to develop a plan that includes regular check-ups, discussions with qualified practitioners who understand or are willing to understand cultural nuances, and exploring alternative therapies if conventional treatments fall short. Emphasizing the importance of being one's own advocate within the healthcare system can't be overstated. Women must feel empowered to question and push back against dismissive attitudes or inadequate care, reinforcing that they know their bodies best and have the right to comprehensive and empathetic health services.

Community awareness and outreach initiatives further emphasize the need for action and engagement at both individual and collective levels. Organizing forums, health fairs, and informational sessions focused on menopausal health can significantly raise awareness and educate communities. These initiatives should aim to include and possibly partner with healthcare professionals who respect cultural contexts, providing a well-rounded perspective that blends medical expertise with lived experience. Such engagements can demystify menopause-related health concerns while promoting an atmosphere where women feel comfortable discussing their symptoms and treatment options openly.

Main Points Recap

Understanding menopause through the distinct lens of Black women's experiences sheds light on how historical, socio-economic, and cultural aspects uniquely shape their journey. This chapter has delved into these complexities, revealing how enduring historical stresses manifest in physical symptoms and emphasizing the importance of equitable access to healthcare and nutrition. By highlighting these challenges, we can better appreciate why tailored approaches are essential for effective symptom management. The resilience embedded within cultural practices and community networks offers significant support, underscoring how collective strength helps balance the scales amidst systemic inequities.

Engaging with culturally competent research and initiatives is key to advocating for improved health outcomes. By fostering environments that respect and incorporate cultural nuances, we empower both individuals and communities to navigate menopause more effectively. Health professionals and wellness coaches play a crucial role here, armed with insights into the specific challenges faced by Black women. Encouraging open dialogue, supporting peer networks, and promoting holistic well-being cultivates an empathetic and inclusive approach. As society progresses towards recognizing the need for diverse representation and personalized care, this chapter serves as a call to action for everyone involved in providing support during this life stage.

Chapter 3: Health Challenges and Self-Advocacy

Health Disparities and Self-Advocacy in Menopause Care for Black Women

Navigating menopause presents unique challenges for Black women, especially when compounded by prevalent health disparities. Menopause is a significant time of change, one that requires a thoughtful approach to manage its complex symptoms effectively. For Black women, these challenges are often magnified by chronic health conditions such as hypertension, diabetes, and obesity, which are more common in this community. These conditions not only add layers of complexity to managing menopause but also highlight the critical need for effective self-advocacy within healthcare settings. The combination of these factors makes it essential to understand the landscape of menopause through the lens of racial and health disparities.

The chapter delves into these pervasive health issues that frequently accompany menopause among Black women, making self-awareness and advocacy crucial. It explores how cultural biases in healthcare can affect treatment and diagnosis, emphasizing the importance of seeking culturally competent care. Chronic conditions like hypertension, diabetes, and obesity take center stage, outlining their impacts on menopausal symptoms and overall health. The chapter also provides insights into strategies for managing these health challenges through diet, lifestyle changes, and collaboration with supportive healthcare providers. By advocating for themselves, Black women can navigate menopause more confidently, armed with knowledge and support to alleviate symptoms while addressing underlying health concerns. Through a compassionate and informed approach, the chapter aims to empower both Black women and those who support them, offering a pathway towards healthier living during this pivotal life stage.

Prevalence of Hypertension, Diabetes, and Obesity

In the landscape of menopause, Black women encounter unique challenges significantly influenced by chronic health conditions such as hypertension, diabetes, and obesity. These conditions are more prevalent within this demographic, underscoring a critical need for heightened awareness and advocacy. This prevalence is not merely a statistic but a living reality that affects daily experiences and impacts overall health. Addressing these concerns begins with understanding the extent to which these chronic ailments permeate lives and their potential consequences.

Hypertension, or high blood pressure, is notably widespread among Black women and poses significant risks if not managed properly. The persistent strain on the cardiovascular system can exacerbate menopause symptoms, leading to severe health outcomes such as heart disease and stroke. Similarly, diabetes, particularly type 2, is more common in Black women, owing partly to genetic predispositions and socioeconomic factors that influence lifestyle choices. This condition disrupts normal bodily functions, affecting everything from energy levels to organ health, compounding the fatigue and mood changes often associated with menopause.

Obesity is another prevalent issue with profound implications during menopause. Excess body weight can amplify hot flashes and night sweats, making everyday life challenging. It also increases the risk of developing additional health problems like arthritis and certain cancers, adding layers of complexity to menopause management. Thus, recognizing the interplay between these chronic conditions and menopause symptoms becomes crucial in mitigating their impact.

Given these compounded health risks, awareness plays a pivotal role in transforming how Black women navigate menopause. Understanding the statistics—not just as abstract numbers, but as indicators of real-world health trends—can empower individuals to take control of their well-being. With awareness comes the opportunity to implement dietary and lifestyle changes that can alleviate symptoms and promote long-term health. For instance, reducing salt intake, engaging in regular physical activity, and incorporating whole foods into one's diet are practical steps toward managing hypertension. Such proactive measures can help maintain balanced blood sugar levels for those affected by diabetes and contribute to healthier weight management.

Understanding these connections sets the stage for informed decision-making, leading to healthier lifestyles that accommodate the intricacies of menopause while addressing chronic conditions. But beyond personal lifestyle adjustments, there's an imperative for culturally relevant resources and strategies tailored specifically to Black women. Collaborating with wellness coaches who understand the cultural nuances and dietary preferences of Black communities can be immensely beneficial. These professionals can offer tailored advice that respects cultural traditions while promoting healthful adaptation.

Guidance in this context extends beyond mere survival through menopause; it involves thriving amidst challenges by leveraging knowledge and resources. Community-based programs and support groups can further enhance this effort, providing spaces where shared experiences foster understanding and encouragement. In these environments, Black women can find solace and strength in shared narratives, gaining insights into managing menopause's complexities.

Access to accurate information and supportive networks empowers Black women to advocate for themselves within healthcare settings. An informed patient can effectively communicate with healthcare providers about specific needs and concerns. This dialogue is crucial for achieving the best care outcomes, as it ensures that treatment plans are holistic and mindful of the unique intersecting factors at play. Advocating for oneself means demanding attention to all dimensions of health, including those often overlooked due to systemic bias or lack of awareness.

Ultimately, the journey through menopause for Black women should not be laden with unnecessary burdens. By shining a light on the prevalence of chronic conditions and their implications, we open a pathway to better health management. Encouraging self-advocacy and fostering a sense of community equips Black women to face menopause with confidence and resilience. As these discussions continue, they pave the way for future generations, ensuring that no woman has to navigate such a transformative period without the necessary support and resources.

Influence of Systemic Healthcare Biases

In understanding systemic biases in healthcare, it's essential to recognize how these disparities have historically affected Black women, particularly during menopause. Systemic biases often contribute to misdiagnoses and inadequate care, underscoring the need for self-advocacy. These biases arise from long-standing stereotypes and misconceptions about Black women's health needs, frequently leading to their symptoms being minimized or ignored.

Healthcare providers may unconsciously perpetuate bias through preconceived notions of pain tolerance and symptom presentation among Black patients, impacting diagnostic accuracy. For instance, the stereotype that Black individuals can endure more pain than others can lead to insufficient treatment of menopausal symptoms such as hot flashes or joint pain. This misconception not only leads to poorer health outcomes but also erodes trust between patients and healthcare providers.

Adding to these challenges are the historical inequalities that linger in modern medicine, continuing to impact health outcomes for Black women. From the days of unethical medical experiments to present-day disparities, the legacy of mistrust has deep roots. This mistrust is further fostered by a lack of representation in clinical trials and medical research, resulting in less information available on how menopause specifically affects Black women. Consequently, treatment options and care strategies remain less tailored to their unique experiences.

It is within this context that personal experiences of discrimination become powerful stories highlighting the necessity of advocacy. Many Black women report feeling that their voices are unheard during medical consultations, which can delay appropriate intervention and worsen health complications. Sharing these experiences can encourage others to be proactive about their health concerns and validate the need for change within the healthcare system.

Such narratives underscore an urgent call to acknowledge existing biases in order to move toward equitable care. By bringing conscious awareness to these biases, healthcare professionals can begin to dismantle the barriers that hinder effective treatment for Black women. Acknowledgment is the first step in cultivating an environment where all patients receive respectful and comprehensive care, regardless of race or background.

Navigating the healthcare system with these biases can be daunting, but there are practical steps that can empower Black women during menopause. One approach involves seeking healthcare providers who are attuned to cultural competence, meaning they are trained to understand and respect diverse cultural backgrounds. Building relationships with empathetic and informed practitioners can make a significant difference in care quality and overall experience.

Additionally, documenting symptoms and preparing questions ahead of appointments can facilitate clearer communication with healthcare providers. Bringing a trusted friend or family member to medical consultations can also provide emotional support and ensure that important discussions are understood and retained.

Moreover, connecting with support groups of other Black women experiencing menopause can offer both solidarity and shared resources. Such communities provide opportunities to discuss common challenges and successful strategies, reinforcing the importance of collective advocacy in the fight against systemic bias.

Strategies for Effective Self-Advocacy

Navigating menopause is a significant life stage, and for Black women, self-advocacy during this period becomes crucial given the unique health disparities they face. By arming themselves with practical strategies, Black women can take charge of their health journey during menopause and ensure they receive the care and understanding they deserve.

First and foremost, assertive communication plays an integral role in enhancing dialogue with healthcare providers. This means confidently expressing symptoms, concerns, and expectations to ensure that their voices are heard and needs are met. An example of assertive communication could be directly discussing any discomfort with treatments or medications, asking clarifying questions, and even seeking second opinions when necessary. A guideline for effective communication techniques includes preparing questions before appointments, maintaining eye contact, and using "I" statements to express feelings and concerns. This approach not only empowers individuals but also fosters a more productive relationship with doctors and nurses, leading to better tailored healthcare solutions.

Knowledge is a powerful tool, especially when it comes to menopause, a phase characterized by complex hormonal changes. Understanding what menopause entails, the potential health impacts, and the specific symptoms one might experience enables informed decision-making regarding treatment options and lifestyle modifications. Women who educate themselves about menopause can critically evaluate the advice they receive, participate actively in treatment discussions, and recognize when symptoms might signal underlying health issues. Utilizing resources such as reputable websites, support groups, and educational seminars can provide insights into managing symptoms effectively and exploring alternative therapies if traditional treatments fall short.

In addition to education and communication, regular health check-ups are fundamental in supporting early detection of any menopause-related issues. Routine screenings and consultations can help monitor key health indicators like blood pressure, cholesterol, and bone density, which often require special attention during menopause. Regular visits create continuity in care, allowing healthcare providers to track any changes over time and adjust treatment plans as needed. For Black women, who statistically face higher risks of chronic illnesses such as hypertension and diabetes, these check-ups are particularly vital. By establishing a consistent schedule for health evaluations, individuals can address concerns proactively and mitigate potential complications early on.

Collaborative planning with healthcare providers further ensures alignment with personal health goals, laying the groundwork for a holistic approach to menopause management. This involves engaging in open discussions about personal health objectives, whether it's maintaining a certain level of physical activity, adhering to a specific dietary regimen, or addressing mental health concerns. By sharing these goals, women enable their physicians to tailor treatment plans that accommodate their lifestyles and preferences. For instance, if a woman aims to manage weight gain—a common issue during menopause—her provider can recommend a balanced diet and exercise plan that aligns with her needs and cultural practices.

To cultivate such collaboration, consider setting up joint meetings with other healthcare professionals or bringing a trusted family member or friend to appointments for additional support. Documenting progress and revisiting health goals regularly also contributes to a dynamic plan that evolves with changing circumstances and experiences.

Ultimately, self-advocacy in menopause care involves a multi-faceted approach: mastering assertive communication, expanding knowledge about menopause, committing to regular health monitoring, and fostering collaborative relationships with healthcare providers. By implementing these strategies, Black women can actively combat health disparities and advocate for the high-quality, personalized care they deserve during this pivotal stage of life.

Embracing these strategies requires courage and commitment, but the payoff is immense. Not only does effective self-advocacy lead to better health outcomes, but it also offers a sense of empowerment and control over one's life journey during menopause. As every woman's experience is unique, it is important to remember that there is no one-size-fits-all solution. Instead, personalization and adaptability stand out as key elements for successful advocacy.

Importance of Culturally Competent Care

In understanding the necessity of culturally competent care, it's crucial to first recognize how it impacts the health outcomes of Black women navigating menopause. At its core, culturally competent care bridges gaps in understanding, promoting trust between healthcare providers and patients. This trust is essential, as it fosters a safe space for discussing symptoms, medical histories, and personal experiences that are deeply intertwined with one's cultural background.

Trust is the foundation upon which effective healthcare is built. When healthcare professionals take the time to understand a patient's cultural context, they demonstrate respect and empathy. For Black women experiencing menopause, this means acknowledging unique stressors and societal challenges that may contribute to their health concerns. By knowing the nuances of cultural influences, providers can offer more personalized and empathetic care, which is often missing in traditional healthcare settings.

Accurate diagnoses and tailored treatment plans naturally flow from an understanding of cultural competence. Menopause symptoms can vary widely among individuals, but when viewed through the lens of cultural sensitivity, healthcare providers can consider important factors such as dietary habits, family medical history, and even traditional remedies that might influence symptomatology and treatment success. For instance, understanding the significance of certain herbs or supplements common in Black cultures can lead to better-informed decisions about pharmacological treatments and lifestyle adjustments.

Furthermore, recognizing the importance of faith, family, and community in a patient's life can inform the approach to treatment. Healthcare providers who practice cultural competence often create a collaborative environment where medical advice is woven with these key aspects, resulting in a holistic approach to care. This ensures not just physical well-being but also emotional and social support during the menopausal transition.

Identifying providers who practice cultural competence becomes a vital step in achieving equitable healthcare. For many Black women, finding a provider who respects and understands their cultural identity can be transformative. Resources like directories of culturally competent practitioners or community recommendations can help in making informed choices. Prospective patients should feel empowered to ask questions about the provider's experience with diverse populations and their approach to culturally sensitive care. Asking these questions can gauge the provider's commitment to personalized and inclusive care.

Guidelines for identifying culturally competent providers include seeking out those who have received training in diversity and inclusion, or who come recommended by community organizations dedicated to supporting Black women's health. Many professional associations increasingly recognize the importance of cultural competence, providing certifications or endorsements that can guide patients in their searches. Additionally, online reviews and testimonials can offer insight into others' experiences and help identify providers who excel in this area.

Beyond individual practice, advocacy for systemic change is crucial in promoting equity within healthcare provisions. Systemic changes ensure that culturally competent care is not just an exception but a standardized expectation across all healthcare services. Advocacy efforts can take many forms, from grassroots community initiatives to policy-driven movements aimed at reforming healthcare systems.

Campaigns advocating for mandatory cultural competence training for all healthcare workers highlight the importance of equipping practitioners with the skills necessary to understand and serve diverse populations effectively. These efforts align with broader healthcare reforms that seek to dismantle systemic barriers contributing to health disparities. By advocating for policies that prioritize diversity in medical training and practice, we can foster environments where culturally competent care is the norm rather than the exception.

Moreover, supporting organizations that lobby for equal access to resources and healthcare improves outcomes for marginalized groups, including Black women experiencing menopause. Community involvement and activism are powerful tools for fostering change, amplifying voices that demand recognition and respect within the healthcare system. Health professionals can also join these initiatives, using their expertise and platforms to raise awareness and promote inclusive practices.

Even though the individual effort is necessary, broader systemic transformation requires a collective push. Collaborating with local community leaders, joining patient advisory boards, or participating in public forums can elevate the conversation around healthcare equity. Advocacy for systemic change is about creating a future where all individuals receive care that respects their cultural identities and meets their unique needs during critical life stages like menopause.

Building a Supportive Healthcare Network

Creating a supportive network during menopause is essential for addressing the unique health disparities faced by Black women. By cultivating connections within healthcare, family, and community, individuals can foster an environment rich in understanding and empowerment.

To begin with, it is crucial to recognize that various roles within one's healthcare network contribute uniquely to support. Family members provide emotional backing, which can be invaluable during the challenging periods of menopause. Open dialogue with loved ones ensures they understand the changes occurring and can offer the necessary encouragement and help when needed. This might include accompanying visits to medical professionals or simply being a sympathetic ear on difficult days. Healthcare providers form another cornerstone of this network, offering professional guidance tailored to personal health needs. They are instrumental in diagnosing symptoms accurately and recommending effective treatments.

Strong relationships with healthcare professionals are pivotal for personalized care. Trust and communication between a patient and their doctor enable detailed discussions about symptoms and ensure treatment plans align with the individual's specific health profile. It is important for health professionals to listen actively and consider cultural factors that impact treatment decisions. Building alliances with empathetic and culturally aware practitioners can lead to better understanding and management of menopause symptoms, creating a smoother transition through this life stage.

To create these alliances, consider openly discussing your specific needs during consultations. Encourage healthcare providers to acknowledge the unique challenges faced by Black women during menopause.

Ask questions about their experience with similar cases and discuss any apprehensions you might have. Bringing family members to appointments can also bridge the gap between clinical advice and home-based supportive care, ensuring everyone involved is informed and aligned in their approach.

Beyond professional healthcare settings, community resources play a vital role in providing additional education and support. Local organizations and groups focusing on women's health can offer workshops, seminars, and discussion forums dedicated to menopause awareness. These platforms not only provide educational opportunities but also allow individuals to connect with others experiencing similar challenges. For instance, attending a local support group could introduce new strategies for managing symptoms while reinforcing a sense of camaraderie.

Community centers, libraries, and even online spaces can host talks or classes led by experts in nutrition, wellness, and mental health, which are particularly beneficial. Utilize these resources to gain insights into managing menopause through dietary adjustments or mindfulness practices suitable for Black women. Accessibility to such programs can be a stepping stone toward achieving holistic well-being, adding layers of knowledge to the support already available from family and healthcare professionals.

Shared experiences within communities foster a powerful sense of belonging and empowerment. Engaging with others who have firsthand knowledge of the struggles associated with menopause creates an invaluable support system. Hearing stories from peers or elder women can be both comforting and informative, offering practical advice alongside moral support. These interactions not only boost confidence but also reduce feelings of isolation commonly experienced during menopause.

Understanding collective strength lies in recognizing and harnessing the wealth of knowledge and resilience among Black women. Traditional practices, cultural norms, and lived experiences come together to form a rich tapestry of support that can guide new generations through menopausal transitions. Establishing intergenerational dialogues within the community promotes the sharing of wisdom and strategies that are grounded in cultural relevance and empathy.

As you navigate this transformative period, remember that involvement in advocacy can serve as a catalyst for change beyond personal care. Supporting initiatives aimed at improving healthcare services for Black women can have lasting impacts on policy and practice. By drawing attention to systemic issues and advocating for equitable treatment options, larger community structures can be influenced, benefiting all those who follow.

Getting involved in local or national advocacy campaigns provides an opportunity to lend your voice to the cause. Collaborate with organizations working towards healthcare equity, attend community meetings, or participate in surveys to highlight the needs of Black women in menopause. Personal experiences can add authenticity and urgency to advocacy efforts, influencing decision-makers to implement positive changes in healthcare policies and resource allocation.

Bringing It All Together

The chapter underscores the critical importance of self-advocacy for Black women facing menopause, especially in addressing health disparities heightened by systemic healthcare biases. It is emphasized that effective self-advocacy includes being well-informed about personal health needs and communicating assertively with healthcare providers to ensure comprehensive care. By mastering these strategies, Black women can significantly influence their healthcare experiences, ensuring their concerns are acknowledged and addressed with cultural understanding and respect. As the chapter explores, this empowerment not only improves individual health outcomes but also strengthens a community-wide movement toward equitable healthcare practices.

Moreover, culturally competent care surfaces as an essential factor in enhancing the menopausal journey for Black women. Healthcare that aligns with cultural identities fosters trust and mutual respect between patients and providers, paving the way for more accurate diagnoses and personalized treatment plans. Connecting with support networks and community resources further enriches this experience, offering both educational opportunities and emotional solidarity. Through collective advocacy and informed choice, Black women can break down barriers within the healthcare system, advocating for recognition and tailored support that respects their unique cultural narratives. Such proactive steps promise a future where navigating menopause is less burdensome and more empowering—both for present-day individuals and the generations that follow.

Chapter 4: The Galveston Diet for Holistic Health

Tailoring the Galveston Diet for Black Women during Menopause

Adapting the Galveston Diet to suit the unique nutritional needs of Black women during menopause is a thoughtful and nuanced undertaking. Menopause presents a myriad of challenges, from hormonal fluctuations to changing dietary requirements, making it essential to find a diet that not only addresses these concerns but also resonates culturally. For Black women, cultural relevance in dietary choices can enhance adherence and make the journey through menopause more affirming and empowering. This chapter delves into the blend of nutrition science and cultural practices, ensuring that the diet is not just effective but also enriching on a personal level.

In this chapter, you will discover how the principles of the Galveston Diet can be tailored to meet the specific health needs of Black women during menopause. The discussion includes practical strategies for integrating culturally significant foods that offer both comfort and nutritional value. Additionally, the chapter explores concepts like nutrient timing and anti-inflammatory eating, providing insights into how these approaches can alleviate common menopausal symptoms. By embracing traditional ingredients and methods alongside modern dietary insights, the adaptation of the Galveston Diet becomes a holistic approach to wellness during this significant life transition.

Principles of the Galveston Diet Explained

The Galveston Diet is a unique approach to nutrition, designed with the specific goal of supporting women as they navigate the changes associated with menopause. By understanding its foundational principles, we can see how it aligns with the needs and cultural contexts of Black women experiencing menopause. At its core, the Galveston Diet emphasizes whole foods and balanced nutrition, aiming for sustainable eating habits that provide long-term benefits.

Whole foods are minimally processed, retaining their natural nutrients, and they form the backbone of this dietary approach. This focus on whole foods helps ensure that the body receives essential vitamins and minerals needed during menopause— a time when nutritional demands may shift. Incorporating vegetables, lean proteins, fruits, and whole grains offers numerous advantages. For instance, leafy greens like spinach and kale are rich in calcium and magnesium, which are vital for bone health. Additionally, lean proteins such as fish or tofu provide necessary amino acids that support muscle mass maintenance, an important factor given the potential loss of muscle tissue during menopause.

However, dietary guidelines aren't one-size-fits-all. Personalization based on cultural preferences can enhance both engagement and adherence to the diet. Celebrating cultural diversity through food allows for the inclusion of traditional elements, which can be nutritious and comforting. For example, the use of collard greens or black-eyed peas in meals not only honors culinary heritage but also contributes fiber and vitamins, promoting digestive health and sustained energy. Encouraging these culturally relevant choices can make sticking to the diet more practical and meaningful, helping individuals stay committed over the long term.

A crucial aspect of the Galveston Diet includes nutrient timing, which can greatly influence metabolism, energy levels, and overall wellness. Nutrient timing refers to the strategic scheduling of food intake throughout the day to maximize metabolic efficiency. Aiming to consume balanced meals earlier in the day can boost metabolism and energy levels, offering support during busy periods. Eating smaller, nutrient-dense meals at regular intervals also prevents blood sugar spikes and crashes, which can help stabilize mood swings commonly experienced during menopause.

Understanding the role of healthy fats is another pivotal component of the Galveston Diet. Healthy fats are essential for reducing inflammation and supporting heart and brain health. Sources such as avocados, nuts, seeds, and olive oil deliver unsaturated fats that aid in the absorption of fat-soluble vitamins like D and E, which are critical for immune function and skin health. Furthermore, omega-3 fatty acids found in fish like salmon can decrease inflammation and improve cardiovascular health, which is particularly significant given the increased risk of heart disease during menopause. Including these fats also supports cognitive health, helping to maintain focus and memory amidst hormonal shifts.

Incorporating these principles into everyday life requires a thoughtful approach, blending dietary guidelines with personal tastes and preferences. Engaging with the Galveston Diet by focusing on whole foods, respecting cultural food traditions, timing meals strategically, and including healthy fats can lead to better health outcomes. Not only does this diet aim to alleviate menopause symptoms, but it also seeks to empower Black women, allowing them to take control of their wellness journey in a way that celebrates and respects their individuality.

Benefits of Anti-Inflammatory Eating

Inflammation is a natural biological response, but it can lead to negative effects when it's chronic. In the context of menopause, also known as the time when women transition out of reproductive age, inflammation can exacerbate common symptoms. These include hot flashes, joint pain, and increased fatigue. For Black women experiencing menopause, considering an anti-inflammatory approach can be particularly beneficial in managing these symptoms. The Galveston Diet, which emphasizes anti-inflammatory foods, offers a tailored solution that meets specific nutritional needs during menopause.

Understanding the impact of inflammation starts with recognizing its role in the body. Inflammation is part of our immune system's defense mechanism. Short-term inflammation plays a crucial role in healing injuries or infections. However, when it becomes chronic due to factors like poor diet, stress, or environmental influences, it can contribute to several health issues. For menopausal Black women, chronic inflammation may intensify symptoms such as insomnia, mood swings, and weight gain. By focusing on dietary changes that minimize inflammation, we can aim for improved symptom management and overall well-being.

Several foods are known for their anti-inflammatory properties, making them essential additions to the Galveston Diet. Incorporating these into daily meals can promote better health outcomes. Leafy greens, such as spinach and kale, are rich in vitamins and antioxidants that combat inflammation. Berries, including blueberries and strawberries, provide essential nutrients and phytochemicals that help reduce oxidative stress. Fatty fish like salmon and mackerel are excellent sources of omega-3 fatty acids, known for their powerful anti-inflammatory effects. Additionally, nuts like almonds and walnuts offer healthy fats and protein while being gentle on inflammation levels.

The introduction of spices such as turmeric and ginger can further enhance this dietary approach. Turmeric contains curcumin, a compound with significant anti-inflammatory benefits, perfect for adding flavor while promoting wellness. Ginger is another powerful spice, often used in traditional remedies, that can soothe inflammatory responses. Regular inclusion of these foods helps not only in alleviating certain menopausal symptoms but also in boosting overall energy and vitality.

Cultural relevance in meal preparation is key for adherence and satisfaction. This involves strategically incorporating anti-inflammatory foods into culturally familiar dishes. Meal prep strategies can be pivotal in making this process efficient and enjoyable. Planning meals ahead of time helps manage portion sizes and ensures balanced nutrition, preventing impulsive food choices that might worsen inflammation. Start by selecting a few core anti-inflammatory ingredients for the week and use them across different meals. A variety of vegetables, lean proteins, and whole grains should form the bulk of your grocery list.

Consider preparing a vibrant salad featuring mixed greens, colorful peppers, avocados, and chickpeas, drizzled with olive oil and lemon juice. This dish could accompany grilled fish seasoned with turmeric and black pepper, combining good taste with anti-inflammatory benefits. Another quick option is a smoothie loaded with berries, leafy greens, and a spoonful of flaxseeds.

Culturally relevant recipes should also have room in the weekly meal plan. This allows connection to heritage while adhering to dietary goals. For instance, substitute regular rice with quinoa or couscous in traditional dishes, or replace heavy sauces with avocado-based salsas. These alternatives maintain the essence of beloved recipes while aligning with anti-inflammatory principles.

Sharing community recipes can empower Black women to explore this dietary approach together, fostering both pride and support. Engaging in communal cooking sessions or recipe swaps can strengthen cultural ties and provide new culinary insights. These gatherings serve as a reminder that food is not just sustenance, but a celebration of culture and identity.

An example of a community-inspired dish might be a hearty gumbo using seafood instead of sausages, with lots of vegetables and spices like cayenne pepper and thyme. Such a dish can remind individuals of familial roots while supporting health objectives. Likewise, exploring Caribbean or Southern motifs with modern twists—like stews enriched with assorted beans and ground provisions—can ensure meals remain nutritionally robust and delicious.

Guidelines for storage and preparation of these recipes are equally important. Making large batches and freezing portions for later can save time and keep the diet consistent. Labeling containers with reheat instructions helps maintain nutrient density and encourages continued consumption of wholesome meals.

Creating Culturally Resonant Meal Plans

In celebrating cultural heritage while adhering to the Galveston Diet, it is essential to explore traditional Black foods and their benefits. These foods not only nourish the body but also strengthen connections to ancestry and culture. For instance, yams, collard greens, and okra have been staples in many African American households for generations. Yams are rich in vitamins C and A, offering immune support and acting as antioxidants.

Collard greens provide an excellent source of calcium and fiber, promoting bone health and aiding digestion. Meanwhile, okra is known for its high vitamin content and potential blood sugar regulation benefits.

By incorporating these nutrient-dense foods into meal plans, women can maintain a connection to their roots while supporting their health. This connection fosters a sense of belonging and comfort, important elements for individuals experiencing menopause. The familiar tastes and aromas create a comforting culinary experience, forging bonds to heritage that may be particularly grounding during this life transition.

Adapting traditional recipes to fit health guidelines without sacrificing flavor or satisfaction requires a thoughtful approach. Many beloved dishes can be adjusted to align with the principles of the Galveston Diet, which emphasizes whole foods and balanced nutrition. For example, traditional fried catfish can be transformed into a healthier option by opting for air frying or baking instead of deep-frying. The crispy texture can still be achieved using a light coating of crushed nuts or seasoned flour alternatives.

Similarly, soul food favorites like macaroni and cheese can be made using whole grain or legume-based pasta, offering more fiber and protein compared to the standard refined pasta. Incorporating vegetables like spinach or kale not only boosts nutritional value but also satisfies taste buds. Substituting lower-fat cheeses or plant-based options can lower calorie intake without compromising the dish's creamy texture. Providing these adapted recipes can empower readers to continue enjoying their favorite meals while taking control of their dietary health.

Balanced macronutrient intake is crucial in managing menopause symptoms effectively. The Galveston Diet can support this balance by focusing on appropriate proportions of carbohydrates, proteins, and fats in each meal. Carbohydrates should primarily come from complex sources such as whole grains, legumes, and vegetables to provide sustained energy and prevent blood sugar spikes. Protein is vital in maintaining muscle mass, especially as metabolism shifts during menopause. Lean sources like poultry, fish, or plant-based options such as tofu and lentils offer valuable choices. Healthy fats, including those found in avocados, nuts, and olive oil, support hormone production and aid in reducing inflammation, a common challenge during menopause.

Combining these macronutrients thoughtfully ensures that each meal provides lasting energy and supports bodily functions. Women in menopause can benefit from prioritizing these balanced meals to cope with symptoms like fatigue and mood swings, contributing to overall wellness and stability.

Family involvement in meal planning presents an opportunity for shared accountability and bonding, enhancing the dining experience. Encouraging family members to participate in planning and preparing meals creates a supportive environment where everyone feels invested in healthy eating. This collective effort nurtures a deeper understanding of both the Galveston Diet and cultural culinary traditions, strengthening familial ties.

By engaging family members, including spouses and children, in conversations about food preferences, dietary goals, and recipe ideas, families can create mealtime routines that reflect joint commitments to health and culture. This collaborative approach also eases the burden often felt by one individual responsible for meal preparation, shifting it to a communal activity where contributions are valued and appreciated.

Shared meal planning sessions can become educational experiences where family members learn about the nutritional importance of certain foods and how they align with traditional practices. These discussions might involve exchanges about historical significance or stories tied to particular dishes, offering opportunities for intergenerational learning and storytelling.

Moreover, cooking together becomes an occasion to teach practical skills and develop a shared legacy of health-conscious eating alongside traditional culinary practices, enriching each participant. Preparing meals collectively allows for flexibility in accommodating diverse dietary needs or preferences, ensuring that each individual's health requirements are met harmoniously within the family structure.

Incorporating Intermittent Fasting

Intermittent fasting has gained recognition as a beneficial approach to health and wellness, particularly during hormonal transitions such as menopause. For Black women navigating this phase, the strategy can be tailored to address specific needs associated with menopause, offering potential relief from symptoms while promoting overall well-being. Understanding the variety of fasting strategies available is crucial for finding what fits best.

Various fasting methods can aid in balancing hormones and managing symptoms like hot flashes, mood swings, and fatigue. Typically, these strategies include the 16/8 method, where one fasts for 16 hours and eats within an 8-hour window, or alternate-day fasting, which involves eating normally one day and consuming minimal calories the next. Such regimens work by influencing insulin sensitivity and growth hormone levels, thereby playing a role in energy regulation and metabolism—critical factors during menopause.

The practice of fasting isn't new; it's deeply rooted in cultural histories that span generations. Traditional fasting rituals, observed in numerous cultures and religions, provide a sense of familiarity and continuity that can be comforting. African cultural practices, such as ancestral reverence through fasting, can be harmoniously aligned with modern intermittent fasting techniques. In doing so, not only are the physical benefits harnessed, but a deeper appreciation for cultural identity and heritage is also fostered.

Blending these traditional practices with contemporary approaches requires understanding both the cultural significance and physiological impacts of fasting. It's about respecting time-honored traditions while making them relevant in modern contexts. This blend can enhance resilience against menopause symptoms, providing a holistic pathway to wellness that resonates on both personal and community levels.

Incorporating fasting into daily life may initially seem challenging, but practical tips can ease the transition. It's vital to start slowly, perhaps beginning with shorter fasting periods and gradually extending them as the body adjusts. Identifying fasting windows that align with one's natural routines—such as skipping breakfast or delaying dinner—can make integration seamless. Staying hydrated and focusing on nutrient-dense foods when breaking a fast ensures that nutritional needs are met despite reduced eating periods.

Listening to the body is essential, as each woman's experience with menopause is unique. Recognizing hunger cues, energy levels, and emotional states will guide adjustments to fasting schedules. Consulting with healthcare providers helps tailor fasting plans to individual health conditions and lifestyle factors, ensuring safety and efficacy.

The role of community support cannot be overstated in enriching the fasting journey. Shared experiences offer encouragement and motivation, helping individuals stay committed. Engaging with family, friends, or local groups fosters an environment where experiences are shared, struggles addressed, and successes celebrated. Community provides collective wisdom and diverse perspectives, making the fasting experience more fulfilling.

Cultural practices intertwined with fasting enhance this communal aspect. Consider organizing group events centered around fasting themes—potluck dinners featuring recipes suitable for breaking fasts or workshops discussing the intersection of nutrition and cultural traditions. These activities bolster a sense of belonging and pride while facilitating shared learning and growth.

Moreover, online communities and social media platforms serve as expansive networks for those seeking broader connection and support. Stories and tips exchanged within these spaces reinforce fasting goals and offer fresh ideas for maintaining engagement.

Foods that Support Hormonal Balance

As Black women navigate the challenges of menopause, maintaining hormonal balance becomes vital for well-being. Key vitamins and minerals play a crucial role in hormonal health during this phase of life. Vitamins D and E are particularly important; Vitamin D supports bone health and mood regulation, while Vitamin E acts as an antioxidant, combating oxidative stress that might exacerbate menopausal symptoms. Magnesium plays its part, too, by aiding sleep and reducing anxiety, which can be especially beneficial when experiencing hormonal fluctuations. Iron is another mineral to keep on the radar, ensuring energy levels remain steady as anemia risks may rise during menopause.

Incorporating these nutrients into daily meals doesn't have to be complicated. Foods rich in these vitamins and minerals include leafy greens, nuts, seeds, and fatty fish like salmon. These are not only easy to integrate into existing diets but also bring added benefits for overall health. Exploring recipes that combine these ingredients with traditional cuisine can add familiarity and comfort while nourishing the body effectively.

Fiber-rich foods serve as allies in achieving both gut and hormonal balance, an area gaining attention for its impact on menopausal health. Traditional grains such as millet, sorghum, and quinoa offer fiber and essential nutrients that help stabilize blood sugar levels, a factor closely linked with hormonal stability. Legumes like black-eyed peas, lentils, and chickpeas also deliver substantial fiber, promoting regular digestion and potentially easing bloating—a common complaint during menopause.

Enjoying these fiber sources doesn't mean abandoning tradition. In fact, incorporating them into beloved dishes can enhance their nutritional profile without compromising taste. For instance, adding chickpeas to stews or using quinoa as a base for salads can introduce variety while keeping meals satisfying and nutrient-packed. The aim is seamless integration, where these foods become staples rather than occasional inclusions.

Managing hormone levels can also be supported by understanding and utilizing anti-estrogenic foods. These foods are instrumental in modulating estrogen activity, offering relief from symptoms like hot flashes. Foods such as flaxseeds, broccoli, and cabbage contain compounds known as phytoestrogens, which mimic or influence estrogen's action in the body, helping maintain balance.

Incorporating these into everyday meals is practical and straightforward. A smoothie packed with flaxseeds and berries, or a side dish of broccoli with garlic, can easily fit into regular meal plans. Understanding these foods empowers women to make dietary choices that align with their body's requirements during menopause, thus actively participating in symptom management.

Indigenous ingredients provide yet another avenue for enhancing health during menopause, celebrating cultural heritage while reaping nutritional rewards. Foods like okra and amaranth, deeply rooted in African culinary traditions, boast health benefits aligned with managing menopause. Okra's high magnesium content can support relaxation and better sleep, while amaranth delivers iron and fiber necessary for sustained energy and digestive health.

Exploring these ingredients opens doors to culinary experimentation, creating excitement and pride in one's heritage while making informed choices about health. Recipes that highlight these foods allow for new interpretations of traditional dishes, blending nostalgia with modern nutritional insights. It fosters a sense of cultural connection, turning meal preparation into a celebration of identity and wellness.

Bringing It All Together

In this chapter, we've explored how the Galveston Diet can be adapted to meet the unique nutritional needs of Black women experiencing menopause. By emphasizing whole foods, respecting cultural food traditions, and strategically timing meals, this dietary approach offers a pathway to manage menopausal symptoms effectively. The inclusion of healthy fats supports heart and brain health, while culturally relevant choices enhance diet adherence. This blend of nutrition and cultural respect empowers Black women, allowing them to take control of their wellness journey during this life transition.

Looking ahead, it's crucial for those seeking to support Black women through menopause—whether healthcare professionals, caregivers, or wellness coaches—to recognize the importance of culturally relevant dietary strategies. Through thoughtful meal planning and embracing traditional foods while integrating modern nutritional insights, we create not only healthier individuals but stronger communities. By celebrating cultural heritage and focusing on balanced nutrition, we're fostering an environment where Black women in menopause can thrive holistically.

Chapter 5: Cultural Connections and Healing Foods

Exploring the Connection Between Food, Cultural Identity, and Health in Menopause

Exploring the connection between food, cultural identity, and health in menopause is a journey that uncovers the profound impact dietary choices can have during this significant life stage. For Black women, traditional foods hold not just nutritional value but a deep sense of heritage and empowerment, offering solace and strength amid hormonal changes. This chapter delves into the richness of cultural cuisine as a roadmap for navigating menopause with grace and resilience. By acknowledging the healing power embedded in ancestral recipes, we open doors to holistic well-being that cherishes both body and soul.

In the following pages, we will explore how specific ingredients commonly found in Black cultural diets can alleviate menopausal symptoms, emphasizing the role of phytoestrogens and anti-inflammatory properties. You'll discover how culinary traditions serve as more than sustenance; they are a bridge connecting generations and a source of shared wisdom. We'll discuss the adaptation of age-old recipes to meet modern health needs without losing their essence, creating a balance between honoring heritage and embracing wellness. Furthermore, the chapter highlights the importance of community engagement, whether through cooking classes or family gatherings, as vital for reinforcing cultural bonds and mental health during menopause. Health professionals will find insights on integrating culturally relevant practices into care plans, while wellness coaches and nutritionists can learn strategies to support their clients effectively. Through these discussions, this chapter aims to inspire Black women to harness the power of their culinary heritage as a catalyst for vibrant health and enduring identity during menopause.

Traditional Foods as a Source of Healing

Traditional foods have long played a medicinal role in the lives of many cultures, and their significance is especially profound for Black women managing menopause. These foods are more than just nourishment; they embody cultural identity and history, which can be empowering and healing during this transformative stage of life. By understanding the science behind these traditional ingredients, one can appreciate their potential benefits.

One of the key components found in traditional diets is phytoestrogens. These naturally occurring compounds mimic estrogen in the body, potentially reducing hormonal fluctuations that lead to symptoms such as hot flashes and mood swings. Foods rich in phytoestrogens include soybeans, flaxseeds, and certain grains. In the context of Black cultural cuisine, ingredients like beans, peas, and nuts also carry phytoestrogenic properties. Integrating dishes made from these elements into daily meals could offer a gentle and natural way to ease menopausal symptoms.

The journey of menopause isn't solely a physical one; it intertwines deeply with emotional well-being. Traditional foods often possess anti-inflammatory properties that not only support physical health but also provide an emotional connection. For instance, turmeric, ginger, and various leafy greens frequently used in African and Caribbean cuisines, hold strong anti-inflammatory effects. These ingredients can combat the chronic inflammation linked to many health issues, further supporting overall wellness during menopause. The act of preparing and consuming these meals becomes a ritual that ties health with cultural identity, offering comfort and continuity.

Recipes passed down through generations hold immense cultural significance. However, adapting these family recipes to incorporate healthier alternatives creates a bridge between heritage and modern health needs. Imagine swapping refined grains for whole grains or using leaner cuts of meat while still maintaining the cherished flavors and aromas. This adaptation not only preserves cultural significance but fosters community support. Sharing modified family recipes allows Black women to navigate menopause with a sense of shared experience and communal strength.

Community plays a crucial role in the healing process. Engaging with elders, who are custodians of ancestral knowledge and culinary traditions, enhances the understanding and usage of these healing foods. Inviting them to cook together not only enriches the palate but also the mind, promoting mental health and reducing feelings of isolation. Elders often hold techniques and insights on ingredients that might otherwise be forgotten. Their involvement becomes pivotal, reinforcing bonds across generations and imbuing the practice of food preparation with stories and meanings.

Guidelines for preserving family recipes in contemporary times become essential here. Initiatives such as community cooking classes or recipe exchange events can empower women to embrace their culinary heritage while making healthier ingredient choices. Such activities create a network of support and learning, where participants share experiences and tips on managing menopause through diet. These gatherings serve as occasions for storytelling and education, fostering deeper connections within the community.

Embracing traditional foods extends beyond individual households. Health professionals and caregivers can benefit from understanding these cultural nuances, helping them tailor advice and care plans to better suit the unique needs of Black women during menopause. Nutritionists and wellness coaches should also advocate for the inclusion of traditional dishes in dietary consultations, recognizing their dual role in providing physiological and emotional sustenance.

To integrate these practices effectively into modern diets, a creative approach is vital. Incorporating traditional spices and ingredients into everyday meals can transform simple dishes into sources of healing and cultural expression. Exploring new variations of familiar recipes helps maintain interest and adherence to a balanced diet, ensuring beneficial nutrients are consistently consumed.

For those experiencing menopause, the journey becomes less daunting when seen through the lens of shared culture and collective wisdom. Traditional foods symbolize resilience and adaptability, offering more than mere sustenance. They provide a sense of belonging and pride, connecting Black women to their roots while encouraging them to embrace change.

Reclaiming Nutrient-Dense Soul Foods

Soul food, beloved for its rich flavors and deep cultural roots, offers more than just comfort; it provides an abundance of nutrients that can be beneficial, especially during menopause. As Black women navigate this significant life stage, understanding the nutritional value inherent in traditional soul foods brings about a shift toward healthier meals without sacrificing tradition or taste.

Firstly, let's delve into the heart of these dishes: the ingredients. Soul foods often incorporate greens, beans, and whole grains—each a powerhouse of essential nutrients. For instance, collard greens are not just a staple of Southern cooking but also a fantastic source of fiber. Fiber is crucial as it supports heart health and reduces inflammation, both important considerations during menopause when hormonal changes can have broader effects on overall well-being. Similarly, legumes and whole grains in dishes like black-eyed peas and cornbread provide protein and complex carbohydrates, assisting in maintaining steady energy levels and satiety throughout the day.

Notably, adapting recipes without losing their essence is a practical approach to enhancing health benefits while keeping the flavor profile intact. Consider substituting turkey for pork in traditionally meat-heavy dishes. This simple swap cuts down on saturated fats, which are linked to increased cholesterol levels and cardiovascular risks—a pertinent health consideration during menopause. The aim here is to preserve the comforting taste and texture soul food is known for, ensuring meals remain satisfying yet nutritionally forward-thinking.

Moreover, maintaining original flavors while subtly boosting nutritional content isn't merely a culinary choice—it's an homage to heritage. Recipes passed through generations hold stories of love, resilience, and creativity. By making health-conscious adaptations, Black women can honor these legacies, safeguarding them for future generations while addressing contemporary health needs. This dual benefit reinforces bonds across families, allowing women to celebrate their heritage with pride and purpose at the dinner table, anchoring family gatherings in both tradition and nutrition.

Food reclamation is another empowering aspect of redefining soul food. Taking control of dietary choices fosters confidence and autonomy. As Black women reassess and reshape their menus, they contribute to health resilience that extends beyond their kitchens. These individual acts of reclamation encourage broader community discussions around diet and wellness, sparking conversations that can lead to collective upliftment and support. It positions food not just as sustenance, but as a medium for empowerment and change. Encouraging dialogue within communities about healthy eating can create networks of shared knowledge and experience, vital for dispelling myths and misinformation about nutrition and menopause.

Creating health-focused versions of classic soul food dishes doesn't mean abandoning tradition—it's a way to enhance and modernize it. Using spices and herbs skillfully, for instance, maximizes flavor without relying heavily on salt or fat, aligning more closely with health guidelines while still delivering the rich taste expected from soul food. This reimagining of recipes serves as a bridge connecting the past with the present, demonstrating that cultural identity and health are not mutually exclusive but rather beautifully intertwined.

Recipe adjustments could also involve incorporating more plant-based elements, leaning towards a diet that embraces diversity and balance. Dishes like sweet potato stew or vegetable gumbo can be made by reducing animal products and increasing the variety of vegetables, providing a means to introduce more vitamins and antioxidants into each meal. These nutrients play a crucial role in managing menopausal symptoms such as hot flashes and mood swings, offering natural relief through diet alone.

Through the act of reclaiming and reshaping soul food, women can engage in meaningful conversations with one another, swapping tips, sharing experiences, and supporting each other. This communal approach not only enriches personal health journeys but creates a collective tapestry of knowledge. It encourages an environment where food is celebrated for its ability to heal, nurture, and connect. As women talk openly about their choices and the benefits they witness, they inspire others to explore similar paths, building a supportive network that champions well-being across different stages of life.

African-Influenced Culinary Heritage

African culinary traditions carry with them a rich legacy of flavor, nutrition, and cultural identity. These elements can be seamlessly woven into contemporary diets, offering profound benefits, especially for Black women navigating the unique challenges of menopause. The base ingredients that form the backbone of many African dishes—such as spices, whole grains, and legumes—not only hold cultural significance but also align perfectly with modern dietary recommendations.

Spices play a crucial role in African cuisine. Their bright colors and robust flavors offer more than just taste; they bring health benefits by providing essential antioxidants and anti-inflammatory properties. Turmeric, ginger, and cayenne pepper are prime examples, each packed with unique compounds that promote overall wellness. Incorporating these spices into daily meals can ease inflammation-related discomforts commonly experienced during menopause, such as joint pain and digestive issues. This subtle integration enhances both the nutritional value and the sensory experience of food, inviting individuals to rediscover and enjoy their cultural heritage on a deeper level.

Whole grains like millet, teff, and sorghum have been staples in African diets for centuries and continue to offer significant health benefits. These grains provide slow-releasing carbohydrates, vital nutrients, and fiber, supporting sustained energy levels and healthy digestion. For menopausal women, maintaining stable blood sugar levels is crucial in managing weight gain—a common concern during this life stage. By incorporating these wholesome grains into meals, Black women can honor their ancestral food practices whilst pursuing modern health goals. Whether transformed into porridge, bread, or added to salads, these grains offer versatile options to enrich the diet while acknowledging cultural roots.

Specific African dishes celebrated for their richness in legumes and grains also contribute to emotional and physical well-being. Take, for instance, traditional stews like Nigerian Egusi soup or Senegalese Thieboudienne, which combine an array of vegetables, beans, and grains. These dishes not only deliver balanced nutrition but also provide proteins and essential vitamins that support hormonal balance and digestive health. The act of preparing and enjoying these meals can foster a sense of comfort and connection, helping to alleviate stress and emotional fluctuations often associated with menopause.

Honoring these culinary practices goes beyond the kitchen. It inspires creativity in everyday cooking, allowing individuals to merge traditional flavors with personal health objectives. This fusion paves the way for playful experimentation in developing new recipes that respect traditional methods while adapting to contemporary tastes and dietary needs. Such innovation empowers women to reclaim their culinary heritage, fostering a renewed appreciation for age-old practices and encouraging lifelong learning and adaptation.

Advocating for these time-tested cooking methodologies encourages a shift away from processed foods, which are frequently linked to adverse health outcomes. Prioritizing whole, nutritious ingredients supports better health and well-being, reinforcing the notion that simplicity in food preparation often leads to more profound nourishment. Community education plays a vital role here, providing tools and resources to help individuals make informed dietary choices rooted in cultural knowledge. Workshops, cooking classes, and community gatherings focused on traditional African cooking can bridge generational gaps, bringing elders and youth together to share stories, skills, and meals.

Establishing a collective understanding of these culinary traditions within communities contributes to holistic health outcomes. It nurtures a sense of belonging and shared purpose, highlighting the importance of food as a means of sustaining not just bodies, but also relationships and identities. Collective efforts can challenge misconceptions about African cuisines, underscoring their place as valuable contributions to nutritious eating patterns globally.

In this journey of culinary exploration, guidelines can serve as helpful companions, guiding integration and adaptation without overwhelming the process. When engaging with culinary legacies and modern applications, it's beneficial to identify core techniques and ingredients that translate well across diverse dietary preferences. Experimenting with portion sizes, seasoning levels, and preparation methods allows for customization, meeting personal and familial tastes without losing authenticity.

For those advocating for African food practices, creating awareness campaigns or educational materials that articulate the health benefits and cultural significance of these traditions can be impactful. Highlighting success stories or testimonials from individuals who have integrated African culinary traditions into their menopausal wellness strategy may inspire others to do the same.

Integrating Food Rituals into Daily Life

Menopause is a significant transition in a woman's life, often accompanied by both physical and emotional changes. For many Black women, the role of food rituals during this period is deeply connected to mindfulness and wellness. Engaging in these rituals not only helps manage menopause symptoms but also strengthens cultural identity and personal well-being. The process of eating becomes more intentional as each meal is seen as an opportunity to connect with one's heritage and foster self-awareness.

Food rituals are more than just the act of consuming a meal; they transform regular meal times into moments of reflection and connection. Mindfulness, when applied to eating, encourages individuals to savor each bite, appreciate the flavors, and consider the journey of the ingredients from the earth to the plate. This practice can make dining a meditative experience, focusing on the present moment and helping to reduce stress, which is particularly beneficial during menopause.

Creating personal meal rituals can be a powerful tool in enhancing emotional health and strengthening relationships. Simple actions, such as expressing gratitude before eating or taking a moment to acknowledge loved ones who contributed to family recipes, can turn meals into celebrations of life's blessings. Gratitude cultivates a positive mindset, promoting well-being and resilience, which are essential during the menopausal transition. Personalizing these rituals allows individuals to reflect their values and traditions, ensuring that each meal is a grounding experience that supports emotional balance.

As we deepen our understanding of celebratory foods within the Black community, it's clear that these dishes serve as more than sustenance—they symbolize unity, culture, and history. Celebratory foods mark important community milestones and personal achievements, acting as a medium through which stories and memories are shared. By embracing these foods, Black women honor their cultural roots while engaging in supportive community practices. Recognizing the significance of these foods enriches cultural appreciation and strengthens bonds among family members and friends, providing an interconnected support network crucial during life's changes.

Mindfulness and gratitude practices around meals extend beyond emotional benefits; they have tangible effects on digestion and satisfaction. Eating mindfully aids digestion by allowing the body time to prepare for the intake of nutrients, resulting in improved nutrient absorption and reduced digestive discomfort. This attentiveness also contributes to noticing fullness cues more accurately, which enhances satisfaction and prevents overeating. The overall joy and pleasure derived from meals increase as one appreciates the effort and love infused into cooking—a notion especially valued in traditional culinary practices.

For those looking to incorporate these ideas into their daily lives, establishing a consistent mealtime ritual is key. Begin with simple steps like setting aside distractions during meals, focusing on the sensory experiences of eating, and taking a moment to express thanks for the nourishment provided. These adjustments can significantly enhance the dining experience, transforming it into a mindful practice that supports mental tranquility and physical health.

Moreover, Black women navigating menopause are encouraged to explore their ancestral food traditions as a way to reconnect with their lineage and nourish their bodies. Many of these foods, prepared in accordance with time-honored customs, are rich in nutrients that may alleviate some menopausal symptoms, such as hot flashes and mood swings. Incorporating these dishes into regular meal plans can fortify a sense of belonging and continuity, bridging past and present through the language of food.

For caregivers, health professionals, and nutritionists serving Black women, understanding the cultural significance of food rituals is crucial. Culturally sensitive dietary advice respects and integrates these cherished traditions, allowing for more personalized and effective care strategies. Recognizing these practices' role in emotional and social well-being ensures that dietary recommendations are aligned with both the physical and cultural needs of Black women during menopause.

Cultivating a Positive Relationship with Food

In navigating the multifaceted journey of menopause, developing a healthier mindset towards food is essential for Black women seeking empowerment and wellness. This transformation in how we perceive and experience food involves embracing love, nourishment, and culture, all pivotal elements that contribute to a more fulfilling life stage.

Understanding food psychologically begins with acknowledging the societal pressures that accompany food choices. From early on, many experience these pressures, often leading to restrictive diets or a negative body image. Shifting the focus from societal expectations to self-compassion can help circumvent these issues. Compassionate self-view promotes acceptance and empowerment by celebrating one's unique culinary heritage rather than conforming to societal standards. Through introspection and mindful eating practices, women can foster positive relationships with food, turning it into an expression of love and self-care.

Nutrition perspectives are crucial as they define individuals' approach to diet during menopause. Emphasizing body nourishment over stringent food restrictions is a powerful shift in thought. By focusing on balance and variety, diets become less about what is excluded and more about what is beneficial. Incorporating nutrient-rich foods from diverse sources ensures comprehensive health benefits. For example, enjoying a blend of leafy greens, whole grains, and lean proteins not only supports physical well-being but also elevates mental health. Such a balanced approach counters the notion that healthy eating must be restrictive, encouraging an enjoyable and sustainable lifestyle.

The celebration of food diversity reshapes narratives around dietary habits. Recognizing and appreciating the rich tapestry of global cuisines fosters cultural pride, enhancing overall well-being. Transitioning from views of restriction to those of enjoyment requires embracing varied ingredients and culinary techniques passed down through generations. Culinary exploration becomes an avenue for maintaining traditional connections while supporting health. Whether it's indulging in a savory gumbo or savoring jollof rice, each dish is a testament to cultural resilience and identity. Celebrating this diversity allows for a deeper connection to ancestry, enhancing emotional and physical health by uniting culture and nourishment.

Support systems play a vital role in reinforcing healthy food relationships and easing the navigation of dietary changes. Community dialogues and shared cooking experiences establish a sense of belonging and understanding. Engaging in conversations about food within social circles encourages the exchange of ideas and personal experiences, enriching knowledge about dietary practices. Cooking together becomes a bonding activity, strengthening ties and creating new traditions.

These interactions nurture a supportive environment where individuals feel safe to explore and share their culinary journeys.

One practical guideline in shifting nutritional perspectives includes creating varied meal plans that incorporate different textures, colors, and flavors. Planning meals with a diverse range of ingredients can encourage exploration and prevent monotony, making nutritious eating an exciting venture. Additionally, participating in community workshops or cooking classes focused on traditional recipes can deepen understanding and appreciation of cultural nuances, providing a richer context for dietary choices.

Implementing support systems might involve forming local groups or joining online forums dedicated to sharing experiences and resources related to nutrition and wellness. These platforms offer opportunities for learning and exchanging tips on culturally relevant dietary strategies tailored for menopause management. Furthermore, inviting friends and family to partake in cooking activities fosters communal bonds and mutual encouragement, making the transition into healthier eating practices enjoyable and collaborative.

Final Thoughts

This chapter has explored how traditional dietary practices can empower and heal Black women navigating menopause. These foods, rooted in cultural identity and heritage, have the ability to soothe physical symptoms like hot flashes while bolstering emotional well-being. By integrating phytoestrogen-rich ingredients and anti-inflammatory spices from African and Caribbean cuisines into daily meals, women can find comfort and continuity in their food rituals. The act of adapting family recipes allows for a balance between honoring ancestors and meeting modern health needs, fostering shared experiences and community strength.

The collective wisdom passed through generations plays an essential role in this journey. Engaging elders to share culinary traditions not only promotes mental and emotional health but also reinforces family bonds and cultural pride. Health professionals, caregivers, and wellness coaches can enrich their understanding by embracing these cultural nuances, crafting more personalized guidance for Black women during menopause. Building on this foundation, communities can organize cooking classes and recipe exchanges to empower women, offering support networks that celebrate both tradition and nutritious living. Through this lens, food becomes a powerful tool in managing menopause, emphasizing resilience, unity, and growth.

Chapter 6: Nurturing Mental, Emotional, and Spiritual Well-being

Enhancing Mental and Emotional Health through Holistic Approaches

Enhancing mental and emotional health through holistic approaches offers a transformative path for Black women navigating the complexities of menopause. As this chapter unfolds, it seeks to address the distinctive challenges posed by this life stage, intertwined with cultural and societal dynamics. These approaches are rooted in understanding the nuanced experiences faced due to historical traumas, systemic inequities, and societal expectations, all of which have influenced perceptions of mental wellness within the community. By adopting a holistic lens, the focus is on integrating culturally appropriate self-care techniques that resonate deeply, providing not just relief from symptoms but fostering empowerment and resilience.

Readers will embark on a journey that highlights the significance of acknowledging mental health disparities and the stigmas that often accompany them. This chapter delves into these issues with sensitivity, shedding light on how enduring stereotypes and misunderstandings can compound the stress and anxiety Black women might feel during menopause. Through exploring various self-care strategies, such as mindfulness, creative expression, nature-based activities, and community support, the discussion encourages embracing these practices as pillars of strength. The ultimate goal is to provide actionable insights and tools that align with personal and cultural values, enabling individuals and caregivers to cultivate an environment where healing and growth are accessible and celebrated.

Mental Health Disparities and Stigmas Addressed

In understanding the mental health disparities faced by Black women, it's essential to look at the historical traumas and societal expectations that have shaped these perceptions. For centuries, Black communities have borne the brunt of systemic inequities and racial injustices. Events such as slavery, segregation, and ongoing racial discrimination have deeply impacted mental health views within these communities. The legacy of these traumas often manifests in distrust towards mainstream healthcare systems and skepticism about mental health interventions, especially when they do not take cultural nuances into account.

Societal expectations further compound these challenges. Black women, in particular, are often subjected to the "strong Black woman" stereotype, which glorifies resilience while ignoring vulnerability. This expectation can deter individuals from seeking help or acknowledging their mental health struggles, reinforcing a culture of silence around emotional pain and psychological distress. Many feel the pressure to appear strong, both for themselves and their communities, which can lead to internalized stigma regarding mental health care.

Cultural narratives play a significant role in shaping perceptions of mental health within the Black community. Often, these narratives perpetuate stigmas rather than encourage understanding and healing. Traditional beliefs may view mental illness as a sign of personal weakness or spiritual deficiency, deterring open discussions or the pursuit of treatment. Furthermore, media portrayals and societal stereotypes can perpetuate misunderstandings about mental health issues, further alienating those who need support.

Addressing these stigmas requires culturally sensitive conversations about mental health resources. It is necessary for these dialogues to acknowledge and respect the unique experiences of Black women. Health professionals and caregivers can foster trust by engaging in active listening and demonstrating empathy, recognizing that each individual's experience is shaped by their cultural context. By creating safe spaces for Black women to share their narratives without judgment, we can begin to dismantle barriers to accessing care.

Education is a crucial tool in advocating for change and improving mental health outcomes for Black women during menopause. Community-driven education initiatives can empower individuals to become advocates for inclusive mental health support systems. These programs should be designed by and for the community, ensuring relevance and cultural sensitivity. They can include workshops, seminars, and outreach events that address mental health from a holistic perspective, integrating both traditional practices and modern therapeutic approaches.

By highlighting personal stories of resilience and providing platforms for Black women to share their experiences, these educational efforts can challenge prevailing stigmas and promote healing. Sharing narratives helps to normalize conversations about mental health and encourages others to seek help without fear of judgment or shame. This community-focused approach not only educates but also builds solidarity, fostering environments where collective healing and empowerment can thrive.

Guidelines are particularly important when promoting culturally sensitive conversations and advocating for change. For culturally sensitive conversations, it is vital to educate caregivers and wellness practitioners about cultural nuances and communication styles that resonate with Black women. Encouraging patience, empathy, and a nonjudgmental approach can build trust and understanding, making mental health resources more accessible and effective.

In the realm of advocacy, guidelines can assist community leaders in developing educational campaigns that address specific mental health needs. These campaigns might emphasize the importance of mental wellness during menopause and highlight available resources tailored to Black women's unique experiences. By using culturally relevant materials and methods, such as storytelling and community gatherings, these campaigns can amplify voices and drive meaningful change.

Techniques for Managing Stress and Anxiety

Navigating menopause can be a particularly challenging time for Black women who might face unique stressors due to cultural, societal, and personal expectations. This subpoint aims to provide culturally relevant techniques to manage stress and anxiety during this transition, offering insights into breathing exercises, creative expression, nature-based activities, and community support as holistic approaches to enhance mental and emotional well-being.

Breathing exercises are a simple yet powerful tool that can considerably alleviate stress by activating the parasympathetic nervous system. This branch of the autonomic nervous system promotes relaxation, slowing down the heart rate, and reducing blood pressure, effectively counteracting stress responses. These exercises can be performed in various settings—whether you're at home, work, or even outdoors. Starting with basic diaphragmatic breathing, which involves deeply inhaling through the nose, allowing the abdomen to expand fully, and exhaling slowly through the mouth, can be highly beneficial. For Black women experiencing menopause, incorporating these exercises into daily routines offers a moment of calmness amid the chaos, serving as an anchor of peace and stability. Engaging in group settings, such as yoga classes that emphasize breathwork, also reinforces a sense of community and collective resilience against stress.

Creative expression is another effective strategy for managing anxiety during menopause. Engaging in arts and crafts provides a therapeutic outlet that allows emotions to flow freely, offering both reflection and release. Whether through painting, drawing, knitting, or even digital storytelling, creative pursuits enable individuals to explore their innermost thoughts and feelings, fostering self-discovery and healing. For Black women, reclaiming these forms of cultural and personal expression can also be empowering, reconnecting them with artistic traditions and narratives that resonate on a deeper level. Organizing regular art sessions or workshops within the community can further enhance this experience, providing a safe space for sharing, learning, and mutual support. The process of creating art can transcend language barriers, speaking directly to the soul, and offering solace and understanding during turbulent times.

Connecting with nature through mindful walks is another method to improve mental well-being and uplift mood. Nature has a natural ability to soothe the mind, reduce cortisol levels—the hormone associated with stress—and enhance overall happiness. Spending time outdoors, whether in a local park or by the sea, presents opportunities to absorb the calming influence of natural surroundings. Taking mindful walks involves being present in the moment, noticing the colors of the leaves, the sound of the wind, and the feeling of the earth beneath your feet. This practice not only grounds the individual but also fosters a greater appreciation for seasonal changes and life's natural rhythms. For Black women going through menopause, these mindful moments in nature offer a reprieve from daily stresses, reminding them of their inherent connection to the world around them. Community walking groups can also be instituted to promote these shared experiences, encouraging dialogue and camaraderie among participants.

Lastly, participating in community workshops can play an essential role in offering shared experiences that reduce stress and strengthen support systems. Workshops centered around topics such as stress management, dietary strategies, and wellness practices tailored to Black women can provide practical knowledge while fostering a sense of belonging and solidarity. These gatherings create environments where women can openly discuss their experiences, share coping mechanisms, and learn from one another. Such communal engagement not only helps in reducing feelings of isolation but also empowers participants through collective wisdom and encouragement. Introducing elements like storytelling, music, or traditional cooking during these workshops can also add layers of cultural relevance and enjoyment, strengthening bonds and inspiring hope.

Role of Mindfulness in Everyday Life

Mindfulness is a powerful tool for enhancing emotional and mental health, particularly during the transformative phase of menopause. This period can bring about a whirlwind of emotions and physical changes that may feel overwhelming. Mindfulness offers a pathway to manage these challenges by emphasizing living in the moment. At its core, mindfulness involves a conscious awareness of the present—paying attention to thoughts, feelings, and sensory experiences without judgment. This practice encourages individuals to observe their internal and external environment with curiosity and acceptance rather than criticism or resistance.

Living in the moment can be incredibly beneficial during menopause when symptoms such as hot flashes, mood swings, and anxiety often arise unpredictably. By focusing on the present, individuals learn to deal with these symptoms more effectively, reducing their intensity and impact on daily life. For instance, when a hot flash begins, rather than reacting with frustration or anxiety, focusing on your breath and acknowledging the sensation without judgment can lessen the perceived discomfort. This approach empowers women to regain control over their responses, fostering a sense of calm and resilience amidst change.

To integrate mindfulness into daily life, practical exercises like mindful eating and listening are recommended. Mindful eating involves paying close attention to the act of eating—savoring each bite, noticing flavors and textures, and listening to your body's hunger cues. This not only enhances the enjoyment of food but also promotes better digestion and nourishment, crucial during menopause when dietary needs might change. Similarly, mindful listening involves fully engaging with those around you. It means being present in conversations without distractions, truly hearing what others say. This practice fosters deeper connections and understanding, enhancing emotional health by reinforcing relationships and communication.

Guidelines for incorporating these practices can help anchor them in everyday life. For example, setting aside specific times during meals to focus solely on the experience, free from television or smartphones, can promote a habit of mindful eating. When practicing mindful listening, try summarizing what the other person has said before responding, ensuring that you have fully absorbed their message. These simple practices can be easily woven into daily routines, gradually becoming second nature.

Beyond individual practices, group mindfulness sessions provide unique benefits by building community bonds and mutual support. Participating in group sessions can offer solace and connection, especially valuable when navigating menopause's isolating aspects. In a group setting, women can share experiences, learn from one another, and cultivate a shared support network. The communal aspect of mindfulness reinforces that struggle is not faced alone, creating a sense of belonging and understanding. Through guided exercises, meditation, or simple discussions, these sessions foster empathy and collective growth, reinforcing emotional bonds and providing a robust support system.

Scientific research further underscores the benefits of mindfulness for both mental and physical health. Studies reveal that regular mindfulness practice reduces stress, improves mood, and enhances overall well-being. On a physiological level, mindfulness can lower blood pressure, improve sleep quality, and boost immune function—essential factors for maintaining health during menopause. Furthermore, the psychological benefits are compelling; mindfulness is associated with reduced levels of anxiety and depression, increased self-awareness, and improved emotional regulation.

For Black women experiencing menopause, mindfulness practice can be an empowering tool. Historically, societal pressures and cultural expectations have influenced perceptions of health and wellness within the Black community. Embracing mindfulness offers a pathway to challenge these narratives by advocating for personal and community healing through intentional practice. By integrating culturally relevant mindfulness practices, such as rituals that honor heritage or incorporate traditional music and dance, women can deepen their connection to both their community and themselves.

Health professionals and caregivers can also benefit significantly from understanding mindfulness's role in supporting Black women through menopause. By recognizing the unique cultural contexts and challenges faced, caregivers can offer more personalized and effective support. Wellness coaches and nutritionists can incorporate mindfulness techniques into their programs, tailoring them to resonate culturally and personally with their clients. This holistic approach ensures that care extends beyond symptom management, nurturing emotional and mental health.

Developing Personal Self-Care Rituals

In crafting personalized self-care rituals, it is essential to start with self-reflection, serving as a cornerstone for identifying unique needs and preferences. This step requires taking a moment of introspection, allowing you to better understand what emotional and mental nurturance means for you personally. Imagine yourself on a quiet morning, sitting comfortably with a journal or simply in thought. Consider what activities bring you joy, calm your mind, and restore your spirit. Think about the times when you have felt most relaxed, content, or empowered. By examining these moments, you reveal patterns about what truly supports your well-being.

This reflective process not only defines basic self-care activities but also personalizes them, ensuring they resonate deeply with your identity and lifestyle. For example, if you find solace in nature, perhaps a weekly ritual could involve a peaceful walk in a nearby park.

Alternatively, if creativity fuels your soul, dedicating time to art or music can be profoundly healing. Through such reflection, we empower ourselves to craft rituals that are not just tasks but sources of genuine comfort and strength.

Incorporating culturally inspired rituals enhances this personalization journey while connecting us to our roots. Engaging in traditional practices, like tea ceremonies, serves as a beautiful way to honor our heritage and infuse daily routines with deeper meaning. Picture preparing a cup of herbal tea, each step—a gentle reminder of traditions shared by generations before us. The aroma, warmth, and vibrant flavors create a sensory experience that transcends ordinary routine, offering a moment of mindfulness and connection to cultural heritage.

Such rituals are more than just individualistic expressions; they act as bridges linking past wisdom with contemporary well-being practices. Culturally inspired rituals also foster a sense of community and belonging, affirming our identities within a broader cultural narrative. They remind us that we are part of something greater, reinforcing resilience during challenging times.

As we explore these aspects, establishing a consistent self-care schedule becomes vital. Regularity transforms occasional indulgences into lasting habits with profound benefits. Consider setting aside specific times each week solely dedicated to nurturing activities. Much like how appointments or commitments are honored with others, treating self-care with similar respect underscores its importance. A straightforward approach might involve marking down self-care times in a calendar, creating a visual commitment to the nurture of mind and body.

Consistency doesn't mean rigidity. There's room for flexibility within a structured framework. Some weeks may allow for extended periods of self-care, while others might require shorter sessions due to life's demands.

What matters most is that these moments are prioritized, regardless of duration. Over time, the regularity of practice instills a sense of stability, reducing stress and enhancing overall wellness.

The journey toward enhanced well-being isn't one we must undertake alone. The role of accountability groups is significant in motivating adherence to self-care practices. Sharing intentions and goals with trustworthy friends or like-minded individuals fosters a supportive environment where encouragement flows freely. These groups can be informal gatherings or structured meetings held virtually or in person.

Imagine meeting regularly with a small circle of women who share similar journeys. In these safe spaces, participants openly discuss challenges, celebrate successes, and provide valuable insights into strategies working in their lives. This collective sharing cultivates both camaraderie and accountability, holding everyone gently yet firmly on their path toward holistic health.

Furthermore, accountability extends beyond physical meetings. With technology's aid, virtual check-ins or message boards create continuous support networks necessary for sustaining motivation. Knowing others stand ready to offer assistance foster reliability, making it easier to maintain consistency even amid uncertainties.

While writing down ideas about participant roles ensures dynamic engagement, maintaining open dialogues without predetermined structures often births creative, unexpected solutions arising organically. Accountability ultimately reminds us we belong within communities invested in personal growth, emphasizing interconnectedness rather than isolation during all stages of this transformative journey.

In establishing personalized self-care routines, understanding how each element integrates seamlessly focuses on incremental changes, allowing evolution over longer periods. Stepping back occasionally offers opportunities for refinement, adapting techniques reflecting current situations, demonstrating fluidity inherent among successful approaches promoting adaptability amidst life transitions.

Utilizing Affirmations and Spiritual Empowerment

In the journey to fostering mental well-being, particularly during significant life changes like menopause, affirmations and spirituality can be profound tools for Black women. The practice of using affirmations is a simple yet potent way to reshape mindsets, promoting self-acceptance and empowerment. By repeating positive statements about themselves and their abilities, individuals can gradually alter their internal dialogue. This shift is crucial because our thoughts significantly influence our emotions and behaviors. For many Black women experiencing menopause, this period of transition can be challenging, with shifts in identity and self-perception. Affirmations offer a path towards embracing these changes with confidence and positivity.

A comprehensive understanding of affirmations reveals that they are more than mere words; they are declarations imbued with power and intention. Research indicates that when individuals consistently practice affirming beliefs, they can experience reduced stress levels and increased feelings of worthiness and competence. For instance, phrases such as "I am strong, capable, and growing every day" or "I embrace my body's natural rhythms and trust its wisdom" serve as gentle reminders of one's strengths and potential.

Alongside the personal practice of affirmations, integrating diverse spiritual practices can greatly enhance emotional resilience and provide comfort. Spirituality is a deeply personal aspect of life, yet it encompasses universal themes of connection, purpose, and transcendence. Many Black women have drawn strength from varied spiritual traditions, whether through prayer, meditation, or ancestral rituals. These practices can provide solace and reflection during menopause, helping individuals navigate the physical and emotional tides of change.

The integration of spiritual practices involves not only personal introspection but also community engagement. Participating in group prayer or meditation sessions, attending religious gatherings, or engaging in traditional ceremonies can foster a sense of belonging and mutual support. Such experiences underscore the interconnectedness of holistic well-being and emphasize the importance of finding grounding within one's community and cultural heritage.

Creating daily affirmation rituals is another essential approach to weaving positivity into everyday life. A structured routine can help solidify affirmations as a habit, making them an integral part of one's day. Consider starting each morning with a moment of quiet reflection, focusing on affirmations that resonate personally. Incorporate these into your daily activities, perhaps by writing them down in a journal, placing sticky notes around your home, or saying them out loud during moments of solitude.

To ensure consistency and efficacy, it's helpful to follow some guidelines. First, choose affirmations that align with personal values and goals. They should be clear, concise, and stated in the present tense to give a sense of immediacy and relevance. Additionally, repetition is key —set aside time daily to repeat affirmations and reflect on their meaning. Over time, this practice can cultivate a mindset rooted in abundance and growth, allowing for easier navigation of life's challenges.

Additionally, sharing affirmations within communities fosters collective empowerment and serves as a reminder that challenges need not be faced alone. By exchanging affirmations, stories, and experiences, Black women can create networks of encouragement and inspiration. Community gatherings, whether in person or virtual, can become vibrant spaces where affirmations are shared and celebrated.

Through storytelling circles or online forums, women can voice affirmations that have supported them, reinforcing a shared commitment to wellness and resilience. These communal exchanges build solidarity and strength, highlighting the importance of collective healing and growth.

Lessons Learned

This chapter has thoughtfully explored the holistic approaches that can significantly impact mental and emotional health for Black women during menopause. We've journeyed through understanding mental health disparities and the stigmas that add layers of complexity to accessing support. By acknowledging powerful societal narratives, we've uncovered how cultural expectations influence individual perceptions of strength and vulnerability. This understanding sets the foundation for employing self-care techniques that are both culturally sensitive and personally empowering. Techniques such as mindful breathing, creative expression, and immersing in nature have been highlighted not just as stress-relievers but as essential tools for fostering well-being and reinforcing community connection.

As we conclude, it's important to embrace the role of education and structured dialogue in dismantling these barriers. Community-driven initiatives and education programs emerge as beacons for change, offering resources tailored specifically to the experiences of Black women. By sharing narratives and promoting culturally relevant mindfulness practices, this approach not only challenges prevailing stigmas but also lays a path for collective healing. For individuals, caregivers, and wellness practitioners alike, the insights in this chapter serve as a call to action to create empathetic spaces where personal empowerment and community resilience can thrive amidst life's transitions.

Chapter 7: Embracing Exercise and Movement

Designing Exercise Routines for Black Women During Menopause

Designing exercise routines for Black women during menopause is an art that requires careful attention to both physical and emotional well-being. This stage of life, marked by hormonal changes, influences how one's body responds to movement and fitness. The goal is to create a harmonious blend of activities that not only address these changes but also spark joy and empowerment. Understanding the unique needs of Black women in menopause is essential, as it allows for crafting routines that are both effective and personally meaningful. By embracing culturally resonant exercises, the journey through menopause becomes not just manageable but enriching, turning exercise into a source of celebration and strength rather than obligation.

In this chapter, we delve into the importance of movement and how it can alleviate many symptoms associated with menopause, particularly for Black women. We explore innovative approaches to fitness, emphasizing cardiovascular health, strength training, and flexibility exercises tailored to maintain bone density and muscle mass while boosting mental health. With a focus on finding joy in movement, culturally relevant and community-based activities are highlighted, showing how they can enhance motivation and commitment. Additionally, we discuss ways to ensure these exercise routines are sustainable and adaptive to individual needs, offering practical guidance on how to integrate rest and listen to one's body to avoid injury. By focusing on creating personalized and empowering exercise experiences, this chapter equips readers with the tools needed to navigate menopause with resilience and confidence.

Importance of Movement in Menopause

Movement is an essential component in the journey of managing menopause symptoms and enhancing overall health, particularly for Black women experiencing this life stage. During menopause, fluctuating hormone levels can lead to a variety of physical symptoms, including weight gain, hot flashes, and joint stiffness. Regular movement not only helps alleviate these symptoms but also boosts general well-being.

Exercise routines during menopause should be thoughtfully crafted to address specific challenges such as reducing the risk of cardiovascular diseases and maintaining bone density. With heart disease being notably prevalent amongst Black women, incorporating regular physical activity into daily life can act as a preventive measure. Simple exercises like brisk walking, cycling, or dancing make the heart pump more efficiently, improving circulation and lowering blood pressure.

Additionally, menopause is often accompanied by decreased muscle mass and increased fat accumulation. Engaging in strength-building activities, such as resistance training with weights or body-weight exercises, can counteract these changes. These routines help in building lean muscle mass, which increases metabolism and assists in weight management—a critical aspect, as metabolic changes can lead to weight gain during menopause.

Moreover, engaging in regular physical activity brings tremendous benefits to emotional and mental health. Menopause can be a tumultuous time emotionally, with mood swings and anxiety being common experiences. Exercise is a powerful tool for stress relief; it releases endorphins, known as "feel-good" hormones, which combat feelings of depression and anxiety. Activities such as yoga and tai chi offer not only physical benefits but also promote relaxation and mindfulness, helping women navigate emotional shifts with greater ease.

For Black women seeking culturally relevant solutions, it's important to find activities that resonate personally. Whether it's joining an African dance class, participating in community walks, or embracing traditional movements, these activities can enrich the exercise experience and strengthen cultural identity. Movement thus becomes a celebration rather than a task—a source of joy that honors individual heritage while promoting health.

Furthermore, social support plays a vital role in maintaining motivation and commitment to an exercise routine. Engaging in group fitness classes or finding a workout buddy can provide accountability and encouragement, making the process more enjoyable. Sharing experiences and successes within a community fosters a sense of belonging and mutual support, which is incredibly empowering.

While engaging in physical activity, it's crucial to listen to your body and adjust routines as needed. Starting with low-impact exercises and gradually increasing intensity ensures that the body adapts without undue strain, reducing the risk of injury. It is always beneficial to consult with healthcare professionals who understand the unique challenges faced by Black women during menopause to tailor exercise programs accordingly.

Addressing Unique Physical Needs

When designing exercise routines for Black women going through menopause, it's crucial to consider several specific physical needs and challenges. Menopause is a natural transition that influences the body in many ways, including hormonal changes that can affect muscle mass, bone density, and overall energy levels. By understanding these factors, we can better tailor exercise programs that promote well-being during this time.

Firstly, let's talk about body mechanics. As women age, maintaining proper posture and alignment becomes increasingly important. Hormonal shifts can lead to muscle and joint changes, so exercises should focus on strengthening core muscles and promoting flexibility. A strong core supports the spine and helps prevent injuries, which is particularly important since menopausal women are at increased risk for osteoporosis. Yoga and Pilates are excellent options for enhancing body mechanics as they emphasize controlled movements and balance.

Another key consideration is joint health. As estrogen levels decrease during menopause, women may experience joint discomfort or stiffness. It's vital to integrate low-impact exercises that protect joints while still providing cardiovascular benefits. Activities like swimming, cycling, or using an elliptical machine can be gentle on the joints while improving heart health. Strength training is also essential as it supports joint function by reinforcing the muscles surrounding them. However, ensure that the routine involves proper form and gradual progression to avoid strain.

Incorporating rest into exercise routines must not be overlooked. Rest is a critical component of any fitness regimen, especially for menopausal women who might experience fatigue due to hormonal fluctuations and sleep disturbances. Balancing active days with rest days allows the body to recover and rebuild. Including activities such as walking, stretching, or meditation on rest days can aid relaxation while keeping the body moving gently.

Awareness of existing health conditions is another factor to consider when planning an exercise routine. Conditions such as hypertension, diabetes, or obesity may pose extra challenges during menopause. It's crucial to work closely with healthcare professionals to tailor exercise programs that accommodate these conditions. For instance, if hypertension is a concern, exercises should prioritize steady aerobic activities and incorporate techniques to manage stress, like breathing exercises or mindfulness practices.

Making Exercise a Joyful Experience

Menopause is a significant transition in a woman's life, and exercise can be a powerful ally during this time. However, the idea of exercising may sometimes feel like an arduous task rather than a source of enjoyment. The goal here is to reshape that perception and empower Black women to find joy and fulfillment in physical activity amid their menopausal journey.

Fun Fitness Activities

Finding pleasure in fitness begins with selecting activities that excite and engage you. It's crucial to explore different types of exercises that resonate personally. Consider dance-based workouts like Zumba or hip-hop dance classes, which can serve as incredible cardio boosters while allowing you to express yourself creatively. Hiking offers a sense of adventure and connection with nature, making it both exhilarating and calming.

For those who enjoy social interactions, joining group classes such as kickboxing, aerobics, or pilates can make routines more enjoyable. Additionally, engaging in sports like tennis or swimming brings diversity to your exercise regimen while offering competitive fun. Remember, it's not just about burning calories but having a good time. Involve friends or family in your activities for added motivation and laughter.

Creating a Personal Fitness Playlist

Music has an undeniable power to uplift spirits and motivate movement. Creating a playlist of your favorite upbeat songs can transform your workout into a lively event. Choose tracks that spark nostalgia or ones with empowering lyrics that fuel your determination. Whether you're walking, cycling, or doing yoga, let the rhythm guide and energize you.

Diverse musical selections can keep your exercise routine fresh and help maintain your focus. Incorporate tunes from various genres and eras to reflect different moods and intensities. Feel free to experiment with new artists or revisit old favorites. As you curate your list, remember it's all about what resonates with you. Let each beat and melody add joy to your steps and moves.

Setting Realistic Goals

Setting achievable goals is essential in maintaining motivation and celebrating progress. Begin by assessing your current fitness level and identifying areas for improvement. Establish short-term objectives that are challenging yet attainable, like adding five extra minutes to daily walks or increasing the weight in strength training sessions.

It's important to track your achievements regularly. Keep a journal or use fitness apps to record milestones and adjustments. Celebrate small victories, whether it's mastering a new yoga pose or completing a full week of consistent workouts. These accomplishments will build confidence and encourage ongoing commitment.

As you reach initial targets, recalibrate and set new goals, ensuring they remain aligned with personal interests and capabilities. This approach prevents burnout and keeps exercise exciting and fulfilling. Remember, every step forward counts towards a healthier, happier self.

Mindful Movement

Incorporating mindfulness into exercises enhances the experience beyond physical gains. Mindful movement involves focusing on the present moment and connecting deeply with your body. Practices like yoga and tai chi are excellent for promoting relaxation, flexibility, and mental clarity.

During workouts, pay attention to your breathing and how your body feels with each motion. Embrace sensations and emotions without judgment, accepting them as part of your journey. This awareness nurtures a positive relationship with your body and encourages self-compassion, especially when coping with menopause's emotional fluctuations.

Integrating meditation or deep breathing exercises before or after workouts can deepen the sense of calmness and satisfaction gained from physical activity. Approach each session as an opportunity for personal growth, balance, and inner peace.

By altering the perspective on exercise from obligation to enjoyment, Black women can cultivate a lifestyle that embraces wellness holistically during menopause. Engaging in activities that spark joy and setting personalized goals support both physical and mental well-being. Balancing the external exertion with internal mindfulness ensures a rewarding and enriching experience.

Maintaining Strength and Flexibility

Incorporating strength and flexibility training into exercise routines is crucial for Black women navigating the transformative phase of menopause. This period of life often brings unique challenges, including changes in muscle mass, joint health, and overall physical well-being, making it essential to adopt fitness practices that address these specific needs.

Strength training serves as a powerful tool in combating the gradual decline in muscle mass that many women experience during menopause. The hormonal shifts, particularly the decrease in estrogen levels, contribute to this loss, making it vital to engage in activities that stimulate muscle growth and retention. By regularly participating in strength-training exercises such as weight lifting, resistance band workouts, or body-weight exercises like push-ups and squats, women can maintain and even increase their muscle mass. This enhancement in muscle strength not only helps in maintaining everyday functionality but also supports bone density, reducing the risk of osteoporosis—a common concern during menopause.

Guidelines are important when embarking on a strength training regimen. It's recommended to start with lighter weights and gradually increase the resistance as strength improves. Aim for at least two sessions per week, focusing on all major muscle groups. It's beneficial to work with a fitness professional who understands the specific needs of menopausal women to create a tailored program that maximizes benefits while minimizing injury risks.

Flexibility training is another key component that can significantly enhance the quality of life during menopause. Many women experience increased stiffness and decreased range of motion during this time due to hormonal changes. Incorporating activities such as yoga, Pilates, or simple stretching routines can help maintain and improve flexibility. These practices not only aid in keeping joints supple but also enhance posture and balance, which are essential for preventing falls and injuries.

A consistent flexibility routine involves incorporating dynamic stretches before workouts to prepare muscles and static stretches afterward to promote relaxation and recovery. Engaging in flexibility exercises three to five times a week can lead to noticeable improvements in mobility and comfort in everyday activities.

Balance training is equally important in an exercise program designed for menopausal women. With age, proprioception—our sense of body position—can diminish, increasing the likelihood of falls. Exercises like tai chi, balance drills, and standing on one leg can fortify this skill. Integrating balance activities into your routine enhances stability and complements both strength and flexibility training efforts.

Creating a comprehensive routine that includes strength, flexibility, and balance exercises requires thoughtful planning. It's crucial to listen to your body and adjust the intensity and volume based on how you feel, ensuring that the routine remains sustainable and enjoyable. Combining these elements not only addresses physical changes but also contributes to mental well-being, providing a holistic approach to health during menopause.

To truly empower Black women during menopause, it's important to recognize and celebrate cultural influences in exercise preferences. Community-based fitness classes that incorporate music and dance familiar to the cultural background can infuse joy and relevance into the workout experience. Finding joy in physical activity fosters consistency, turning exercise from a task into an enriching part of daily life.

Moreover, engaging with support networks, whether through group classes or online communities, can provide encouragement and motivation. Sharing experiences and progress with others who understand similar challenges can further enhance the commitment to maintaining an active lifestyle.

Incorporating Cardiovascular Workouts

Cardiovascular exercises are invaluable, especially for Black women navigating the transition of menopause. Menopause is a time of significant change, and maintaining heart health becomes crucial. Cardiovascular workouts, by boosting aerobic capacity and improving circulation, play a vital role in fostering robust heart health. They help mitigate risks associated with cardiovascular diseases, prevalent among Black women due to genetic predispositions, lifestyle factors, and socio-economic challenges. By regularly engaging in cardio activities, such as walking or dancing, individuals can significantly lower their blood pressure and cholesterol levels, contributing to a healthier heart.

The physical benefits extend beyond heart health. Cardio workouts enhance overall fitness, increasing stamina, energy levels, and endurance. This not only makes everyday tasks easier but also enriches life by enabling active participation in activities previously considered strenuous. Moreover, improved lung capacity from consistent cardiovascular exercises leads to better breathing and more efficient oxygen use by the body. The holistic improvements offered by these activities make them ideal for those experiencing menopause, which often brings about fatigue. By committing to regular cardiovascular routines, Black women can combat this fatigue effectively, regaining vitality and vigor.

Finding joy in movement through a variety of fun cardio exercises can transform the perception of workouts from a chore to an empowering activity. It's essential to incorporate diversity to keep exercise routines both enjoyable and sustainable over the long term. Options like dance classes, group aerobics, or cycling provide opportunities for social interaction, an added benefit that promotes emotional well-being. Participating in community events or fitness groups can add a layer of culturally relevant support and encouragement, enhancing motivation. Additionally, mixing different activities prevents monotonous routines and engages different muscle groups, contributing to comprehensive physical development.

Guidelines for variety encourage experimenting with different forms of cardio to identify what resonates most. Classes in African dance styles or other culturally significant movements not only enrich the soul but also maintain engagement and foster a sense of cultural pride and identity. Exploring rhythmic movements set to music integrates tradition with contemporary exercise, resulting in a pleasurable and rewarding experience that extends beyond mere physical fitness.

Equally important is understanding the frequency and duration necessary for these exercises to be effective. Health professionals recommend at least 150 minutes of moderate-intensity aerobic activity each week. Divided into manageable sessions, this translates to around 30 minutes on most days. However, flexibility in scheduling can cater to personal preferences and lifestyles. Some may find joy in longer sessions over fewer days, while others may prefer shorter bursts of activity more frequently. Consistency is key, and listening to one's body helps tailor these activities to individual needs, ensuring sustainability and continued growth in fitness levels.

Adopting guidelines for monitoring progress is invaluable in maintaining motivation and ensuring effectiveness. Tracking improvement in endurance, heart rate recovery, or even mood changes post-exercise provides tangible evidence of progress. Utilizing wearable technology or simple pedometers can aid in keeping track of daily steps, offering a sense of accomplishment and encouraging continuous effort. Reflecting on how these exercises impact emotional and physical well-being fosters a holistic approach, validating the comprehensive benefits derived from cardiovascular routines.

Black women experiencing menopause face unique challenges, and recognizing this is fundamental in crafting supportive exercise regimes. Empowerment through education about the benefits specific to cardiovascular workouts allows for informed decisions regarding health and wellness. This knowledge equips them to prioritize self-care, balancing responsibilities while dedicating time to improve their quality of life. Understanding and embracing these benefits is instrumental in cultivating a mindset geared towards health and longevity.

Moreover, healthcare providers and caregivers should appreciate these distinct needs and advocate for personalized cardiovascular programs. By acknowledging cultural and physiological aspects, they can offer guidance that aligns with Black women's lived experiences. Educational workshops or resources aimed at spreading awareness can bridge gaps, facilitating access to appropriate fitness advice and support systems.

Concluding Thoughts

This chapter has explored the importance of creating exercise routines that cater specifically to the unique needs of Black women during menopause. It emphasized movement as a vital component not only for physical health but also for emotional and mental well-being. Tailored fitness strategies help address challenges like heart health, bone density, muscle retention, and weight management while offering joy and cultural connection through activities like dance or community walks. By prioritizing fun in exercise and setting realistic goals, Black women can transform these routines into enjoyable experiences rather than burdensome tasks.

Moreover, incorporating strength, flexibility, and cardiovascular training ensures a comprehensive approach to wellness. This chapter highlights the critical role of social support and healthcare guidance in maintaining motivation and preventing injuries. By celebrating cultural heritage and finding joy in movement, exercise becomes an empowering tool to navigate the complexities of menopause. These insights are meant to guide Black women, their health professionals, and wellness coaches in fostering a lifestyle that embraces both physical vigor and mental tranquility amidst the journey of menopause.

Chapter 8: Celebrating Wisdom and Empowerment

Celebrating Wisdom and Empowerment

Celebrating wisdom and empowerment during menopause involves embracing the journey with confidence and pride. For many Black women, this phase of life is a significant and natural transition that can lead to profound personal growth. Menopause is often misunderstood solely as an end to fertility, yet it presents an opportunity for exploration, introspection, and transformation. It invites women to redefine their lives with resilience and self-acceptance, extracting lessons from past experiences to build a vibrant future. By approaching menopause with adaptability, there is a world of possibilities for prioritizing personal needs and desires, ultimately transforming this stage into one of empowerment and renewed self-discovery.

In this chapter, readers will delve into uplifting perspectives that celebrate the accumulated wisdom gained through menopause. By acknowledging the unique cultural narratives and familial histories that shape each woman's journey, a deeper sense of pride and identity emerges. The chapter offers insights into adapting dietary and lifestyle choices to enhance well-being, emphasizing holistic health that addresses both physical and emotional dimensions. Additionally, the text explores how storytelling and intergenerational mentorship within communities serve as powerful tools for education and empowerment. Finally, by connecting menopause with historical context and cultural reflections, this chapter fosters solidarity and support among Black women, highlighting the significance of shared experiences in viewing menopause not as a loss, but as a continuation of life's rich tapestry.

Uplifting Final Thoughts and Encouragement

Menopause is a natural stage of life, one that signifies not only change but also profound growth and self-reflection. For Black women experiencing menopause, embracing this transition as an opportunity for personal development can transform the experience from one of trepidation into one of empowerment. This stage is often misunderstood solely as the end of fertility, yet it is so much more—a new chapter inviting exploration, introspection, and the chance to redefine one's life.

Understanding menopause as a time for self-reflection fosters an environment where accumulated wisdom is celebrated rather than overlooked. As Black women, acknowledging the unique cultural narratives and familial histories that enrich your journey through menopause can bring about a deeper sense of pride. This phase invites you to look inwardly, encouraging a mindset where the rich tapestry of experiences—both past and present—can be woven into a vibrant outlook on the future. Just like any transformative period, menopause offers valuable lessons about resilience, patience, and self-acceptance, helping to build a bridge toward the person one is becoming.

By viewing menopause through a lens of adaptability, one can feel empowered to prioritize personal needs and desires. During this time, embracing flexibility and revisiting lifestyle choices becomes crucial. Whether it's adopting wellness practices that emphasize nutrition or exploring mental health strategies that promote emotional well-being, tailoring these choices to fit individual and cultural contexts can lead to a more fulfilling experience. Flexibility in this approach encourages the prioritization of holistic health, considering both physical and emotional dimensions. By doing so, menopause is transformed into a powerful journey of self-discovery and empowerment.

The historical context surrounding menopause provides further insight into how older generations have navigated these changes with grace and confidence. Learning from the experiences of elder family members and community leaders can offer invaluable guidance. In many African cultures, menopause has been regarded as a sacred passage, marking the elevation of women into esteemed roles within their communities. These perspectives transform menopause into a symbol of wisdom and leadership, offering a blueprint for navigating the complexities of change with trust in one's strength.

Moreover, history emphasizes the importance of storytelling and oral traditions in passing down knowledge and support. Engaging with these stories allows for a recognition that while the physiological process remains quite universal, the journey of each woman is distinct. Sharing experiences in culturally relevant ways—whether through community gatherings or intergenerational conversations—enhances understanding and builds solidarity among Black women experiencing menopause. It underscores the significance of creating safe spaces where experiences are acknowledged, respected, and celebrated.

Acknowledging the diversity of experiences during menopause helps foster a positive mindset prepared to embrace the upcoming journey. The challenges faced during this time can often highlight accumulated wisdom, showcasing the depth and breadth of personal growth over the years. Each story of overcoming hardship adds another layer to the understanding of what defines strength and resilience. It's essential to recognize and appreciate these moments, cheerfully celebrating the legacy of fortitude established by those who came before, while continuously working towards crafting one's own narrative.

An attitude of curiosity and openness to adaptation allows the menopausal journey to remain dynamic and empowering. By understanding the body's evolving needs, and choosing to listen and respond compassionately, Black women can navigate menopause with increased clarity and empowerment. Developing a personalized approach to wellness that aligns with one's beliefs and values reinforces the notion that menopause is a time for self-compassion and empowerment, not deficiency or loss.

Celebrating the Wisdom Gained in Menopause

The journey through menopause is not merely a biological transition; it carries the promise of profound wisdom and insight. This phase of life offers invaluable lessons that illuminate paths to greater clarity and understanding, especially for Black women navigating both personal and cultural landscapes. In embracing these changes, women find opportunities to reassess and redefine their life goals and values, often with newfound perspective and clarity.

Through menopause, many discover an enhanced focus on what truly matters. This period becomes a natural time for reflection, allowing women to distill their desires and priorities from the noise of everyday life. Such introspection can lead to a deeper understanding of one's core beliefs, paving the way for setting purposeful and intentional paths forward. Whether it involves pursuing long-held dreams or redefining relationships, menopause can be a catalyst for positive transformation and alignment with true self-identity.

Confronting the symptoms and challenges that arise during menopause also serves as a testament to resilience and character building. The physical and emotional hurdles encountered during this time demand a level of strength and endurance that, once embraced, reveals inner fortitude. For instance, managing hot flashes, mood swings, or fatigue often requires adapting to new wellness routines and support systems. In doing so, many women develop coping strategies that enhance their overall well-being. These experiences are particularly empowering as they highlight the capacity to endure and thrive despite adversity.

Such resilience is further amplified by adopting dietary and lifestyle practices tailored specifically for menopause, oftentimes embracing culturally relevant solutions found within Black communities. For example, incorporating traditional foods known for their health benefits into daily meals can provide both comfort and nutritional support. Additionally, exploring holistic wellness practices, such as mindfulness and yoga, can alleviate symptoms and contribute to a balanced lifestyle, reinforcing health and vitality.

Moreover, menopause provides a platform for advocacy and mentorship, where women become guides for younger generations. Sharing personal stories and experiences not only nurtures community bonds but also aids in demystifying menopause for those who may face it in the future. This act of storytelling becomes more than just sharing anecdotes; it transforms into a powerful tool for education and empowerment. Young women gain insights into potential challenges and solutions, fostering a culture of openness and preparedness.

Mentorship extends beyond family circles, influencing broader societal perspectives. Women transitioning through menopause are uniquely positioned to influence policies and practices within healthcare settings, ensuring they cater sensitively to the needs of Black women. By actively participating in discussions about health and wellness, these advocates can push for research and resources that address specific cultural and physiological considerations.

Cultural reflections play a crucial role in enriching the menopausal journey, offering unique insights that connect individuals to their roots and communities. Menopause can serve as an entry point to explore and embrace cultural traditions related to womanhood and aging. Rituals and celebrations acknowledging this life stage can reinforce a sense of identity and belonging. Engaging with heritage and folklore not only fosters understanding but can transform menopause into a shared experience characterized by honor and reverence rather than stigma.

The ways in which different cultures frame and celebrate menopause can offer solace and strength. For instance, some African societies view it as a passage into esteemed elderhood, underscoring the respect and authority gained through life experience. Recognizing these narratives encourages a shift away from negative stereotypes associated with aging, promoting a mindset of appreciation for the life stage's inherent wisdom and grace.

In modern contexts, acknowledging cultural insights helps bridge individual backgrounds with wider community connections. Incorporating these perspectives into support networks enriches collective understanding and enhances solidarity among women experiencing menopause. Events and gatherings focused on cultural expressions can provide spaces for mutual support and learning, where knowledge and traditions are honored and preserved.

Ultimately, the transformative wisdom gained through menopause highlights the richness of this journey. It is a time filled with potential for growth, advocacy, and connectedness. By embracing the depth of experiences offered, women emerge with stronger, clearer visions for their lives and communities. This wisdom moves beyond personal growth, influencing future generations and reshaping societal views on aging and womanhood.

Call to Action for Adopting the Galveston Diet

Embracing menopause with confidence can be a transformative experience, and the Galveston Diet offers an empowering way to enhance well-being during this significant stage. By making small, manageable dietary changes, women can seamlessly integrate the Galveston Diet into their lives, making the transition both practical and effective. Often, the thought of overhauling one's diet can feel daunting, particularly when faced with the myriad changes that accompany menopause. However, beginning with simple adjustments like incorporating more anti-inflammatory foods such as leafy greens, berries, and fatty fish into daily meals can provide a solid foundation. By gradually introducing these changes, women can slowly build momentum toward a healthier lifestyle without feeling overwhelmed.

Understanding food labels and nutrient content allows women to make informed dietary choices, which is pivotal in taking control of health during menopause. Knowing what each label signifies can demystify the process of selecting healthy options, preventing unintentional consumption of ingredients that could trigger symptoms. For example, becoming adept at identifying hidden sugars or unhealthy fats empowers women to choose alternatives that support their overall health. This shift towards informed decision-making can foster a sense of control amidst the physical changes experienced during menopause, reinforcing the idea that knowledge truly is power.

One of the most enriching aspects of integrating the Galveston Diet is the opportunity to connect with others through shared experiences. Sharing meals with family and friends not only strengthens relationships but also provides an open platform for discussing various dietary strategies. These conversations can serve as a source of encouragement and inspiration, motivating individuals to stick to their goals. Participating in community cooking classes further extends this camaraderie, allowing women to collectively learn new recipes and techniques suited for the Galveston Diet. These classes offer much more than culinary skills; they nurture a supportive network where women can exchange tips, share successes, and even failures, creating a sense of solidarity. Such interactions can alleviate feelings of isolation and reinforce the notion that this journey need not be a solitary one.

Engaging in continuous learning about nutrition can have far-reaching benefits, invigorating one's approach to diet during menopause. Staying curious and informed about nutritional advancements opens the door to an ongoing discovery process. It encourages women to refine their diet continually and adapt to what feels best for their changing bodies. For instance, exploring how different foods react with their personal chemistry can lead to custom-tailored eating plans that align closely with individual health needs. This dynamic cycle of learning and adaptation ensures that women remain proactive participants in managing their health.

Practical steps are essential for successfully implementing any new diet. Incorporating guidelines into daily routines, like meal prepping or setting weekly goals, can significantly enhance adherence to the Galveston Diet. Creating a meal plan for the week, based on available seasonal produce, reduces the stress of deciding what to eat each day while ensuring a consistent intake of nutritious foods. Another useful strategy is maintaining a food diary to track eating patterns and identify areas for improvement. Over time, these practices not only fortify discipline but also illuminate positive trends in mood and energy levels directly tied to dietary changes.

Empowerment through informed choices is another vital element. Educating oneself about the origins and benefits of each food item enhances mindfulness in eating habits. Understanding the importance of nutrients like Omega-3 fatty acids, which help reduce inflammation, or antioxidants, which can combat stress-related aging, becomes second nature. Equipped with this knowledge, individuals can select foods consciously, aligning them with specific health objectives linked to menopause, such as reducing hot flashes or boosting metabolism.

Community engagement plays a crucial role in sustaining motivation and enthusiasm towards dietary goals. Organizing regular meetups or potluck dinners centered around Galveston Diet-friendly dishes helps keep the momentum alive. These gatherings act as informal support groups where participants can discuss challenges, celebrate milestones, and exchange practical advice, all while uniting over shared culinary creations. Additionally, leveraging technology to form online communities or join existing forums can broaden access to diverse opinions and support, reaching women who may not have local peers interested in similar dietary pursuits.

Continuous learning about nutrition should ideally be viewed as a lifelong commitment rather than a temporary phase. As scientific research evolves, staying abreast of the latest findings can spark curiosity and adaptive changes in dietary habits. Subscribing to nutrition-related publications, attending workshops, or following credible experts on social media can provide valuable insights. This persistent quest for knowledge

not only aids personal growth but also ensures that
women remain equipped with the most effective tools to
navigate health during menopause and beyond.

Strengthening Community Bonds and Support

Creating a supportive network for women navigating
menopause begins with safe spaces where open
discussions about challenges can flourish. These havens
foster emotional relief, allowing women to express
themselves freely without judgment. In environments
where understanding is the norm, individuals can share
their stories, fears, and triumphs over menopausal
symptoms. This sharing not only lightens personal
burdens but enhances collective wisdom. Safe spaces
cultivate trust, which is essential for meaningful
connections. As women engage in heartfelt exchanges,
they build a tapestry of experiences that inform and
nurture each other.

Guidelines for establishing these safe spaces are crucial
for fostering an atmosphere of respect and empathy. It's
important to ensure that all voices are heard, and
discussions remain constructive. This can be achieved by
initially setting ground rules emphasizing confidentiality,
active listening, and mutual respect. Encouraging regular
meetings and offering diverse discussion topics can also
help maintain engagement and interest.

Organizing peer-to-peer support groups further
strengthens these community bonds. Women find
comfort in knowing they are not alone, and these groups
act as forums for sharing insights and strategies for
coping. They serve as a platform for learning, where
personal experiences provide valuable lessons that
textbooks often overlook. Within these gatherings,
lasting friendships form, rooted in shared understanding
and support.

Guidelines for these groups emphasize inclusivity and flexibility. Meeting formats should accommodate various needs, whether in person or online, ensuring broader access. Peer-led initiatives can promote more authentic and relatable interactions. Inviting guest speakers occasionally can provide additional perspectives and expertise.

Community events, like workshops, bring dynamism to these networks. Such events invite dialogue on menopause from diverse angles, drawing in newcomers and expanding circles of support. Workshops focused on wellness practices, such as yoga or nutrition, not only educate but empower attendees to take proactive steps in managing their menopause experience.

To effectively deliver these workshops, clear guidelines involving planning and execution are beneficial. Collaborating with local organizations or health professionals can enrich content and attract participants. Planning engaging and interactive sessions ensures deeper involvement and learning opportunities. Continuous feedback from attendees can help refine and enhance future events, making them even more impactful.

In our technologically advanced world, leveraging online resources can significantly broaden geographical outreach. Digital platforms offer invaluable opportunities for women to access information and connect with others globally. Online forums, social media groups, and webinars create virtual communities that transcend physical boundaries, allowing shared knowledge to benefit from international perspectives.

To navigate the vast digital landscape, guidelines can steer users towards credible and beneficial resources. Suggestions include promoting validated websites, encouraging participation in moderated groups, and recommending reputable webinars. Educating users on digital literacy can enhance their ability to discern reliable information, ensuring that their journey through menopause is informed and empowered.

Continued Journey of Empowerment and Health

In embracing menopause as a vital component of a continuous journey toward empowerment and holistic health, we find an opportunity to redefine and uplift. This period is not just about physical changes; it's also an invitation to deepen our understanding, reshape our thinking, and embrace new ways of living.

Lifelong learning plays a crucial role in this transformative phase. Continuing to educate ourselves about menopause allows us to stay informed on the latest research and health practices that affect our well-being. This proactive approach extends beyond individual benefit; it encourages community growth as shared knowledge becomes a powerful tool for unity. For example, participating in workshops or reading about newer dietary recommendations can equip you with insights that might help alleviate symptoms such as hot flashes or insomnia. Staying informed means actively seeking out resources that address the unique cultural contexts of Black women, ensuring that advice is relevant and empowering.

Moreover, adopting a holistic approach to health during menopause is essential. Our wellness is not limited to the physical realm. It encompasses mental, emotional, and spiritual dimensions, each interwoven to maintain balance. Engaging in practices like meditation, yoga, or spiritual reflection can enhance mental clarity and emotional resilience, providing grounding amidst change. Nutritional awareness, perhaps through culturally attuned diets, supports physical health, while engaging with creative outlets nurtures the soul. By harmonizing these aspects, we nurture a comprehensive sense of health that respects all facets of our being.

Visualizing empowered futures post-menopause is another key aspect of this journey. Envisioning what life can look like beyond menopause helps set goals and fosters positive outlooks. This act of visualization can be particularly powerful because it transforms abstract hopes into tangible aspirations. Whether it's pursuing a new career, rekindling a passion, or traveling, envisioning these futures provides motivation and framework for action. This practice empowers us to see past immediate challenges and focus on long-term fulfillment.

Encouraging intergenerational learning and activism is vital in creating inclusive pathways for dialogue and empowerment. Sharing experiences across generations enriches our understanding and highlights diverse narratives around menopause. These interactions serve as bridges to wisdom, offering lessons from those who have navigated similar journeys with grace and strength. Organizing community events or casual discussions between younger and older women can spark conversations that debunk myths, cultivate solidarity, and inspire collective activism. Such efforts promote a broader acceptance and celebration of menopause as a natural stage in life rather than a stigma-laden process.

It is crucial to underscore that these elements are not isolated; they are interconnected threads weaving a richer tapestry of menopause experience. The commitment to lifelong learning inspires others to join in collective wisdom-seeking. A holistic health approach ensures we are supported, mind, body, and spirit. Visualization directs our energies towards future possibilities, while intergenerational exchanges ground us in present realities, imbued with the narratives and strengths of those before us.

This journey, while deeply personal, is enriched by community support and shared wisdom. For many Black women, finding culturally resonant solutions during menopause isn't just beneficial—it's essential. Therefore, exploring methods and practices that honor cultural identities and experiences is fundamental to feeling empowered. Health professionals and caregivers must also recognize these needs, adapting their approaches to provide more nuanced, effective care.

Through commitment to these principles, black women can find empowerment within themselves and their communities as they navigate menopause's challenges and triumphs. This transformation isn't just about managing symptoms; it's about embracing a new chapter with enthusiasm and respect for oneself. This perspective shift reframes menopause not as an ending but as a continuation of life's vibrant journey—a step forward into a myriad of opportunities waiting to be claimed.

Concluding Thoughts

As we conclude this chapter, it's evident that menopause is not just a phase but an opportunity for renewal and empowerment. By embracing menopause with confidence, Black women can transform this life stage into a period of profound personal growth and self-discovery. Recognizing the wisdom accumulated over time enables women to redefine their values and priorities, focusing on what truly matters. This chapter has highlighted the importance of culturally relevant strategies that resonate with individual experiences, advocating for a personalized approach to health and wellness. By integrating these tools, women are encouraged to look beyond the physical changes and appreciate the journey toward a more enriched life.

Furthermore, sharing experiences within communities fosters solidarity among those navigating similar paths. It's crucial for women to connect with one another through storytelling and mentorship, creating supportive networks that enhance understanding and empathy. When healthcare professionals and caregivers acknowledge the unique cultural contexts and needs of Black women during menopause, it enriches the care provided and strengthens community bonds. Through continued education, holistic practices, and collective wisdom, menopause becomes a celebration of identity and resilience. Embracing this transformation with pride allows women to confidently step into a new chapter, paving the way for future generations to experience menopause as a natural, empowering part of life's journey.

Conclusion

As you turn the final pages of this book, I invite you to pause and reflect on the extraordinary journey you've been on. Menopause is a transition—a natural and powerful chapter in the story of every woman's life. For Black women, it holds even deeper layers, entwined with cultural richness, unique challenges, and unparalleled strength. It's a juncture that calls for celebration, understanding, connection, action, and anticipation.

Your journey is distinct, marked by experiences that are solely yours to navigate. Menopause does not diminish your essence; rather, it symbolizes growth and transformation. It is crucial to acknowledge that each moment, each change you undergo, contributes to an ever-evolving tapestry of resilience and wisdom. Imagine yourself as a mighty oak tree, standing tall against the winds of time. With every season, there's both beauty and continuity. In the same vein, menopause allows you to cultivate inner wisdom, adding layers to your strength with each year.

Furthermore, understanding menopause from a culturally attuned perspective empowers you with invaluable insights into your health and well-being. Specifically, Black women face unique physiological nuances during menopause that require your attention and respect. By equipping yourself with knowledge— about dietary approaches, lifestyle changes, and holistic practices—you are arming yourself with a vital toolkit. Knowledge becomes your ally, transforming how you experience this period and enabling you to advocate for yourself fiercely when navigating healthcare systems. Grasping these nuances means you're no longer sailing through uncharted waters, but confidently steering your course with clarity and purpose.

In the heart of this transformative journey lies the irreplaceable value of community and shared experiences. There's an inherent power in sisterhood, in gathering strength from shared stories and mutual support. As you traverse this path, remember that you're part of an expansive network of Black women who understand exactly what you're going through. They hold stories similar to yours, hearts that beat in resonance with yours, and arms open wide in empathy and solidarity. This is your circle of strength and sanctuary—a place where you can embrace both the joys and struggles of menopause. Here, in the warmth of community, confidence flourishes and empowerment takes root.

Moreover, taking active steps towards health ownership is a profound act of self-love and determination. The Galveston Diet and other wellness practices presented in this book are more than just guidelines—they're invitations to nourish your being. Today is a new day full of promise. By choosing to savor meals that nurture both body and soul, you begin a deeply personal journey toward reclaiming your health. Every choice you make echoes with empowerment, each small step forging a path to wellness and recognition of your infinite worth. You are steering your own health narrative, crafting a story of vitality and renewal.

And indeed, as you stand on the brink of this new chapter, embrace the future with unwavering confidence. Menopause is neither a halt nor a detour; it is an opening to a fresh voyage brimming with potential and transformation. Think of a phoenix rising resiliently from the ashes, stronger and more magnificent than before. Allow this analogy to guide you as you envisage your future—not as an end—but as a proliferation of beginnings, each offering opportunities for growth, exploration, and fulfillment.

Embrace the power within you to transform adversity into opportunity, solitude into community, and transitions into triumphs. Let this period in your life be defined not by constraints or loss but by unprecedented freedom and possibility. Revel in the myriad colors of your journey. Know that you stand on the shoulders of countless ancestors, wise women who have walked paths paved with challenges and victories. Their legacy is one of resilience, grace, and an indomitable spirit. You too carry this legacy forward.

Explore the potential waiting to blossom in every corner of your life. Whether it's embarking on new adventures, nurturing passions forgotten amidst the bustle of routine, or pursuing purposes yet undiscovered—it's all within reach. Standing strong with newfound wisdom, you possess the tools to chart an exhilarating course across uncharted terrain. With each step, let hope and curiosity be your companions, assuring you that possibilities are endless and that every layer of experience enriches your life's canvas.

May this book serve as a beacon of understanding, companionship, and inspiration as you continue your journey. Your story is one of strength, vibrancy, and boundless potential. Embrace it wholeheartedly. Stand tall and proud, ready to embrace all the wonders that lie ahead. The world awaits your courageous spirit.

This moment, this stage in your journey, is truly remarkable. Celebrate your uniqueness, harness the power of knowledge, lean on your sisters, take control of your health, and face the future with confidence. Each decision you make, every relationship you forge, and all the dreams you dare to pursue will shape a future radiant with promise. So rise, resilient and inspired, into this new beginning, for it's only the start of a beautiful chapter filled with discovery, empowerment, and joy.

www.ingramcontent.com/pod-product-compliance
Lightning Source LLC
Chambersburg PA
CBHW051105250726
48656CB00001B/483

9 7 9 8 3 4 4 0 1 2 2 1 6